Nursing and Women's Labour in the Nineteenth Century

T0252722

This book presents a new examination of Victorian nurses which challenges commonly held assumptions about their character and motivation. Nineteenth-century nursing history has, until now, concentrated almost exclusively on nurse leaders, on the development of nursing as a profession and the politics surrounding registration. This emphasis on big themes, and reliance on the writings of nursing's upper stratum, has resulted in nursing history being littered with stereotypes. This book is one of the first attempts to understand, in detail, the true nature of Victorian nursing at ground level.

Uniquely, the study views nursing through an economic lens, as opposed to the more usual vocational focus. Nursing is placed in the wider context of women's role in British society, and the changing prospects for female employment in the high Victorian period. Using St George's Hospital, London, as a case study, the book explores the evolution of nurse recruitment, training, conditions of employment and career development in the second half of the nineteenth century. Pioneering prosopographical techniques, which combine archival material with census data to create a database of named nurses, have enabled the generation – for the first time – of biographies of ordinary nurses.

Sue Hawkins' findings belie the picture of nursing as a profession dominated by middle-class women. Nursing was a melting pot of social classes, with promotion and opportunity extended to all women on the basis of merit alone. This pioneering work will interest students and researchers in nursing history, the social and cultural history of Victorian England and women's studies.

Sue Hawkins is a researcher at Kingston University, UK.

Nursing and Women's Labour in the Nineteenth Century

The quest for independence

Sue Hawkins

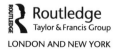

Routledge
Taylor & Francis Group

LONDON AND NEW YORK

First published 2010
by Routledge
2 Park Square, Milton Park, Abingdon, Oxon OX14 4RN

Simultaneously published in the USA and Canada
by Routledge
711 Third Avenue, New York, NY 10017

Routledge is an imprint of the Taylor & Francis Group, an informa business

First issued in paperback 2012

Typeset in Baskerville by Wearset Ltd, Boldon, Tyne and Wear

British Library Cataloguing in Publication Data
A catalogue record for this book is available from the British Library

Library of Congress Cataloging-in-Publication Data
Hawkins, Sue, 1956–
 Nursing and women's labour in the nineteenth century : the quest
for independence/Sue Hawkins.
  p. ; cm.
 Includes bibliographical references.
 1. Nursing—Great Britain—History—19th century. 2. St. George's
Hospital (London, England)—History—19th century. I. Title.
 [DNLM: 1. Nurse's Role—history—England. 2. History, 19th
Century—England. 3. Women's Rights—history—England.
4. Women, Working—history—England. WY 11 FE5 H394n 2010]
 RT11.H39 2010
 610.7309421—dc22   2009040661

ISBN13: 978-0-415-55169-4 (hbk)
ISBN13: 978-0-415-53974-6 (pbk)
ISBN13: 978-0-203-85446-4 (ebk)

For Andrea, David and Joan

Contents

Illustrations

Tables

Pen portraits of nurses

Acknowledgements

When I first started work on the research which led eventually to this book, I was not sure where it would lead. I thought I would be writing a history of one nursing department in a period when nursing was experiencing great upheaval; and the main focus would be the impact of the professionalization movement. But as I dug deeper into the wonderfully rich archive at St George's Hospital, I was drawn more and more to the women who were working there. Who were they, I wondered? Why had they ended up nursing, and why at this hospital? What choices did they have? What was it like to be a nurse in Victorian times? The secondary literature addressed these questions only tangentially, and dated from the 1980s. The focus of my research shifted. I was determined to find a way of uncovering these women's lives, and saving them from the stereotype they had been forced into.

I should say I am not, and have never been, a nurse. It is a constant question I face when meeting colleagues for the first time. My original education was in science, and I worked for 20 years on the periphery of the pharmaceutical industry, before being drawn back to academia through an MSc in History of Science, Technology and Medicine. That led to a life-changing decision – to become a historian.

This project has brought me into contact with a community of historians, of all disciplines, and a world I had no idea existed. So many people have played a part in this book's coming to life.

I am tremendously grateful to Kingston University and, in particular, to Dr Christopher French (then Director of the Centre for Local History Studies) and Kath Start (then Deputy Dean of the Faculty for Health and Social Care Sciences) for awarding me a bursary to pursue my doctoral studies, without which this would not have been possible.

I also to need acknowledge the help and support I have received from a host of friends, colleagues and organizations – too many to mention by name, but one or two deserve special thanks. Marina Logan-Bruce and Nallini Thevakarrunai, Librarian and Archivist, respectively, at St George's Hospital Medical School Library (now both retired), were amazingly helpful in giving me unfettered access to their archive. Nick Baldwin (archivist at Great Ormond Street Hospital) provided similar access to the records there. I must also acknowledge the extremely important support I received from two networks of colleagues, The UK Centre for History of Nursing and Midwifery (at Manchester University) and the Women's History Network. Their importance, in terms of the support they offer to new historians to test their ideas in a supportive environment, cannot be overstated.

But my greatest thanks go to my supervisor, and good colleague, Dr Andrea Tanner, without whose support (and patience) this would probably never have happened. I met her at the archive at Great Ormond Street, volunteering on a project to digitize Victorian admission registers, and her enthusiasm and energy for history infected me. We worked up the original idea for the nursing project and we have been working together ever since. She has been an inspiration on this project, cajoling me when I lost momentum, painstakingly reading draft after draft, and providing too many lunches to number. This book is dedicated in great part to her support.

The book is also dedicated to an old friend, Joan Murphy, sadly no longer with us. Joan (who was suffering from breast cancer) and I would meet occasionally, and over a bottle of wine we would put the world (and our lives) to rights, fantasizing about what we would do if things were different. Joan never got the chance to put her dreams into action, but she gave me the courage to take the plunge, leave my office job, and dare to do something new.

Finally, I have to thank unreservedly my very patient and long-suffering partner, David Hawkins, who has been on as painful a journey as I have, in the incubation of this book and my transformation from office worker to academic researcher. His support has been invaluable and has sustained me through some long hours in the study, reminding me that there was a world outside that I should venture into occasionally.

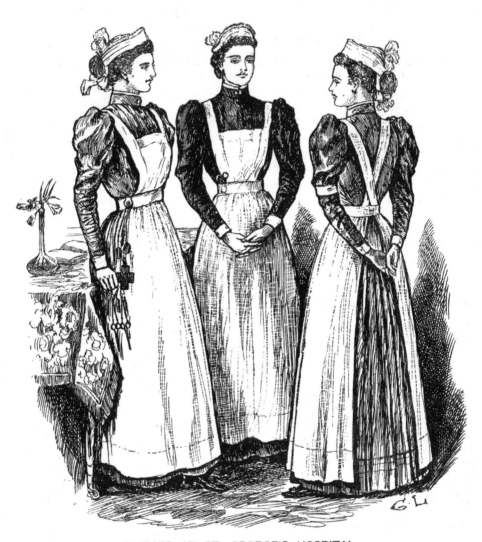

NURSES AT ST. GEORGE'S HOSPITAL.

Plate 1 Nurses at St George's Hospital, *c.*1890s. From *The Hospital (Nursing Mirror Supplement)*, 15 June 1895. Courtesy of *Nursing Times* (reproduced by the British Library Reprographics Unit).

Introduction

Constructing new nursing and a new history of nursing

The history of nursing in England is a young subject. Until the late twentieth century, it was dominated by Whiggish accounts of nursing's relentless progress from an occupation dominated by old and destitute widows to the scientific profession it presents today. Pursued, in the main, by enthusiastic amateurs (often nurses or ex-nurses), nursing history has been dominated by hagiographic accounts of nineteenth-century reformers, chief among whom was Florence Nightingale (Woodham-Smith 1950; Pavey 1938). Until very recently, despite its obvious connections to the changing role of women in society and, more specifically, to women as workers, its history has been discussed without any reference to such themes. Shifts in historical thinking (such as the rise of social history in the 1960s and 1970s, and the emergence of labour history, women's and gender history) passed it by and it continued to be the domain of heroic self-congratulation (Evans 2000). Perhaps, as Celia Davies has suggested, its history suffered as a result of nursing being almost exclusively populated by women (Davies 1980). On the surface, there were no power struggles between the sexes for gender historians; neither could they focus on heroic fights for the recognition of women's right to practise, as nursing was regarded as a naturally female task. Further, there appeared to be no opportunity to study the development of a body of knowledge, as nursing could lay claim to no such unique and cohesive collection through which it defined itself (Davies 1980).

More recently, these assumptions have been challenged, and today nursing history has been placed in a wider context, opening up questions about its relationship with medicine, and how it came to be regarded as the subordinate discipline. The politics of nursing has taken centre stage in these new histories, but studies of the nature of the women who chose to become nurses continue to be elusive. This book will argue that the development of nursing can only be properly understood if more focus is brought to bear on the lives of the women who worked on the wards. It will use one London hospital, St George's, as a case study, to follow the development of a nursing department in the second half of the nineteenth century in detail. The results, which are discussed in the context of the wider subject of women's work in late nineteenth-century England, challenge commonly held assumptions about the reform of nursing in the nineteenth century.

Revisiting the rewriting of nursing history

Detailed historiographies of nursing history now preface all major works on the subject, and illustrate how far the discipline has evolved since the days of Pavey and her glorification of Nightingale. Sociologist Brian Abel-Smith broke the domination by amateur historians with his 1960 book, *A History of the Nursing Profession*. The book's major themes centred on 'the structure of the profession, on recruitment, on terms and conditions of service ... [describing] the activities and rivalries of the professional associations and trade unions which have represented or tried to represent nurses' (Abel-Smith 1960: xi). It has been hailed as the starting point for a new type of history of nursing, displaying objectivity, situating nursing in the context of society at large, and abandoning hagiography (Borsay 2006). Nevertheless, even he fell somewhat in thrall to the Nightingale myth, counterpoising Nightingale's 'charm' against Ethel Fenwick's 'uncompromising' and 'opinionated' approach in his summation of the registration debates (Witz 1992).[1] As a result Abel-Smith dismissed the registration debate as a 'battle for status conducted against a background of rampant snobbery and militant feminism' (Abel-Smith 1960: 67).

Despite the success of Abel-Smith's book, it was 20 years before any new nursing histories emerged. The questions he posed, regarding the nature of nursing and the experience of being a nurse, remained unanswered.[2]

In 1980, a group of nurse historians, under the editorship of another sociologist, Celia Davies, produced a collection of essays which finally took up Abel-Smith's call, and posed new questions of nursing's history. Davies called for an academic vigour previously lacking, urging her contributors to be critical of nursing history's historiography and its methods (Davies 1980). As a result of this collection, several important themes in nursing history emerged, including the rise of nursing as a profession; the origins and nature of relations between doctors and nurses; and the introduction and development of nurse education. In addition, new methodologies were also introduced, pioneers of which included Kathleen Williams and Christopher Maggs.

To this point, most nursing history had been based on the uncritical use of evidence left by nineteenth-century nurse reformers. In 'From Sarah Gamp to Florence Nightingale', Williams questioned whose accounts of nursing's development should be believed, underlining the importance of examining motive among contemporary commentators. Using two accounts of the rise of modern nursing, both written in 1897, she illustrated how interpretation of events can be coloured by the writer's perspective (Williams 1980). Margaret Breay was a pro-registration late nineteenth-century nurse. Her Whiggish account, which appeared in the *Nursing Record*, attributed the rise of modern nursing to the work of influential nurse leaders, starting with Elizabeth Fry, deftly moulded by Nightingale, and resulting in the science-based, education-led profession she recognized as nursing at the end of the nineteenth century. The other writer was a doctor who asserted that the development of the modern nurse was based on well accepted medical practice, and had been guided throughout by the medical profession. Unlike Breay, he was not comfortable with the new focus on nurse education or associated attempts to establish a nursing organization independent of the medical profession.

Who is right? This is not necessarily the best question to ask, and is certainly difficult to answer without knowing the background of the two authors, or the times in which they were writing. The doctor had adopted the protectionist position typical of his profession at the time, concerned that medical authority would be challenged by an autonomous nursing organization. His view of the history of nursing echoed his view of the relationship between medicine and nursing. Miss Breay, on the other hand, was a supporter of registration and the faction within nursing which demanded autonomy from the medical profession. Her view gave nurses the controlling hand in the profession's development.

By selecting accounts from both sides of the professional and gender divide in this way, Williams was able to analyse her sources for signs of bias, and thereby better understand the dynamics of the dispute (Group and Roberts 2001). This critical reading of contemporary nineteenth-century texts is rarely seen in earlier accounts of nursing history, and marked a new approach to its study.

While Kathleen Williams urged nurse historians to review contemporary Victorian accounts of nursing with a new-found critical eye, other methodologies were also emerging. Christopher Maggs chose to examine the subject 'from below' rather than from the perspective of the profession's elite (Maggs 1980).[3] Using hospital employment records as his main source, he challenged assumptions about the nature of Victorian nurses and nursing; and discovered that, contrary to the popular 'heroic' image, the nurses in his study did not measure up to this ideal (Maggs 1980). As with Williams' work, Maggs' investigations at a local level led him to challenge wider assumptions about Victorian nursing. He expanded on the theme in his book, *The Origins of General Nursing*, in which he set out to address the gaps identified by Abel-Smith, especially, 'what it was like at different times to nurse' (Maggs 1983: xi). Unlike previous studies, Maggs' work was based on 'the experiences of the nurses themselves, rather than on the leadership or on reformers of the profession', thereby hoping to address the 'historiographical imbalance' in much of nursing history (Maggs 1983: xi). His work is further marked out from earlier nursing histories by its extensive references to Victorian working women, placing nurses firmly in this category, rather than that of ministering angels. For possibly the first time, the lives of ordinary nurses came under the microscope and Maggs attempted to understand their motivations by combining data from archival sources with material from journals and novels.

Maggs' approach enabled him to ask a series of questions not previously raised: why did women choose nursing above other occupations which were opening up to female employees; did nursing really become an occupation for the middle classes, or was this an ideal which did not coincide with reality; did nursing develop into a career rather than an occupation to be taken up *in extremis* only, and (if so) how did this happen?

As a result of Davies' book and Maggs' work, a growing number of researchers have responded to the call to look at nursing history anew, basing their research on local studies of individual institutions.

Carol Helmstadter has written extensively on the origins and impact of Victorian nursing reforms on London teaching hospitals, and other historians have made use of nursing records to examine the changing profile of nurse recruits at a variety of hospitals (Helmstadter 1993a, 1993b, 1994, 1996, 2001; Wildman 1999). Likeman's study of University College Hospital (UCH), and Simnet's study of St Bartholomew's (Bart's) are examples of this. Their findings, which challenge assumptions about the class structure of end-of-the-century nursing, are discussed in depth in Chapter 2 (Likeman 2002; Simnet 1986). Jane Brooks added to this debate with her study of nursing at St Thomas' Hospital and Leeds General Infirmary, using a similar approach (Brooks 2001).

As the number of local studies proliferate, the reality of the 'modern' nurse as promoted by Victorian nursing reformers becomes less clear. Both Simnet and Likeman have shown that middle-class women were entering nursing by the 1890s, but the work of Brooks and Simnet also suggests that working-class women were not being banished. These mixed results indicate the potential pitfalls of 'history from below': of drawing too broad a conclusion from the study of individuals or small communities, and failing to interpret them in a wider context (Postan, 1971; Tiller 1998; Tosh 2006). Likeman, for instance, failed to discuss the possible impact on her findings of the fact that nursing at UCH was carried out by a sisterhood.[4] Paucity of data in local studies, or non-contiguous data runs, also render trend analysis problematic. However, these difficulties should not discourage further local studies from being undertaken. Even if results are difficult to interpret they can still challenge the integrity of messages being delivered by nurse reformers at the time. Further work on the careers of ordinary nurses, which is one of the chief objectives of this book, will aid the understanding of class structure and supposed prejudice within Victorian nursing.

In 1987, a follow-up to Davies' book was produced under the editorship of Maggs, in which he proclaimed, 'We are witnessing an exciting era in nursing and nursing history, and the tide of new writings looks set to become a flood' (Maggs 1987: 1). One of the common threads of this collection was the development of nursing as a profession, and this has become the dominant theme in nursing history in recent years, returning to Abel-Smith's work on the politics of nursing reform. Maggs' own evocation of 'nursing history from below' has subsequently been lost in the rush to contribute to the 'professionalization project', as Helen Sweet has described this branch of nursing history (2007: 571). The registration debate, where source material is plentiful, may have proved the more attractive option, compared to the prospect of sifting through diverse sources searching for scraps from which to rebuild ordinary nurses' lives.

Anne Marie Rafferty's work on the development of nursing is typical of the dominant discourse from late twentieth-century historians, in works which sweep across the decades from the mid-nineteenth century to the foundation of the National Health Service in 1948 (Dingwall *et al.* 1988; Rafferty 1996). Rafferty contextualizes her arguments in a wider social context, drawing support from the history of education, women's history and gender studies. But by situating them primarily within the registration debate, she inevitably focuses on the nurse leaders and their personalities, rendering the ordinary nurse almost entirely absent from analysis.[5]

Historians have also taken Williams' lead, questioning some of the long-held tenets of traditional nursing history, through the critical analysis of published materials. Nightingale's reputation had been viciously attacked by Lytton Strachey in the early twentieth century, but she continued to hold an unassailable position in the history of nursing until the 1980s, when the mythology surrounding her finally came under scrutiny (Strachey 1918 [2003]). Francis Smith's *Florence Nightingale: reputation and power* (1982) and Monica Baly's *Florence Nightingale and the Nursing Legacy* (1986 [1997]) presented critical appraisals of her contribution to the development of modern nursing. These two works generated a torrent of outrage from Nightingale supporters, indicating the difficulty of challenging traditional interpretations of cherished personalities. Smith's 'debunking of the Nightingale myth' was described by Anne Witz as a 'vicious misogynous tirade', while Monica Baly was branded a revisionist by Ann Bradshaw for questioning the effectiveness of her training school (Witz 1992: 131; Bradshaw 2000).[6] Despite their reception, such works legitimized the critical analysis of Nightingale's role in the development of modern nursing, to nursing history's gain.

Similar analytical techniques have also been employed to challenge the 'old' and 'new' nurses myth, best characterized by the opposing images of Sairey Gamp (the irresponsible old nurse in Dickens' *Martin Chuzzlewit*) and a Nightingale Nurse (a disciplined, chaste young woman). Traditional interpretations have accepted these images at face value – 'old' nurses were ignorant and ill disciplined, in complete contrast to the 'new' nurses. Anne Summers – in another landmark contribution to nursing history – was possibly the first to question the use of the Sairey Gamp image as representative of nursing pre-Nightingale (1989).[7]

Her article, 'The Mysterious Demise of Sarah Gamp', raised several important historiographical points: that the history of nursing before the Crimea had been all but ignored, that it was dominated by a history of hospital nursing, and that contemporary accounts should be examined with care. Questioning the traditional image of pre-reform nurses, she pointed out that during the first half of the nineteenth century most sick people, in all classes of society, were cared for in the home, often by domiciliary nurses working independently of the medical profession. Is it plausible, she asked, that these nurses were, as a body, uniformly disreputable and inadequate? (Summers 1989). Yet this is what the Gamp–Nightingale dichotomy implies. Her analysis of the origins of the Sairey Gamp myth has produced new insights into the relationship between the professions of medicine and nursing, and the motivations of both in relation to nursing reform. Domiciliary nurses, she argued, posed a real threat to the medical monopoly, and the Sairey Gamp figure was used by doctors to discredit such women: 'It was not so much because she was ignorant or vicious that the doctors wished to eliminate her practice, as because she had strong opinions and a large clientele of her own' (Summers 1989: 385).

Nurse leaders used the image to draw stark contrast with the new hospital nurse, who was portrayed as 'uniformed, thoughtful, poised and sober' (Summers 1989: 382). They, too, were fearful of the independence demonstrated by domiciliary nurses, which rendered them difficult to control. Summers' work on domiciliary nurses has highlighted the importance of identifying and querying Victorian stereotypes of nurses and doctors, and of investigating perspectives other than those of nursing's reformers.

It is strange to think that nursing history could be studied without reference to gender, but such has been the case for most of the twentieth century. In 1978, Eva Gamarnikow discussed nursing in such terms, proposing that nurse leaders purposely used gendered arguments to construct a role for women in hospitals which did not threaten the existing male hierarchies. As she explained: 'The doctor/nurse relationship became the man-father/woman-mother relationship and effectively was subsumed under the rubric of female–male relations' (Gamarnikow 1978: 111). A silence followed, and by 1991, clearly frustrated that this theme had not been pursued by fellow feminists, she developed her own arguments further. Nurses and their leaders, she contended, were not passive victims, but had deliberately used such ideologies to construct an occupation specifically for women, led by women. To her, this strategy was not 'a limited or restrictive action, but an enabling one' (Gamarnikow 1991: 111).

Gamarnikow suggested that the lack of engagement in nursing history by feminist historians probably resulted from the imagery of 'passivity, self-sacrifice, devotion and subordination' which suffused it. Lacking the dramatic qualities of the suffragettes or the rebellious nature of Lancashire mill workers, nursing's associations with 'patriarchally constructed femininity', she argued, most likely appalled them (Gamarnikow 1991: 110). Similar arguments have been made about the lack of attention paid by feminists to the history of women's role in the domestic life of families. Leonora Davidoff and Catherine Hall have argued that 'Domestic affairs, cooking, eating, house-cleaning, have been avoided [by historians] as both trivial and unhistorical' (Davidoff and Hall 2002: xxxiii).

The only major feminist contribution to nursing history to appear between Gamarnikow's two discourses was produced in 1985 by feminist historian, Martha Vicinus. Her influential book on single women in Victorian society contained a chapter on the rise of nursing as a respectable profession, which continues to be widely referenced today (Vicinus 1985). Unlike Gamarnikow, she was not as optimistic about the nurse reform project. Rather, she argued that nursing, unlike other occupations opening up to middle-class women at the time, 'grappled with creating a sphere for women amid a male world', but failed to establish an independence from it (Vicinus 1985: 119). In her view, nurse leaders became obsessed by the politics of state registration, and as a result they ignored the plight of ordinary nurses, failing to fight for, 'shorter hours, better pay, and adequate pensions' (Vicinus 1985: 120). Echoing Abel-Smith from 30 years earlier, she accused nurse leaders of 'class prejudice and sexism [which] collided to create a weak secondary occupation rather than the strongly united corps of women so celebrated in [their] pronouncements' (Vicinus 1985: 120).

Similar lack of interest in nursing history has been shown by labour historians. Despite Mick Carpenter's contention that the history of nursing is simply, 'one chapter in the history of labour', few labour historians have discussed it (Carpenter 1980: 125). Lee Holcombe's *Victorian Ladies at Work* provides a narrative account of the development of nursing as an occupation for middle-class women during the latter half of the nineteenth century (Holcombe 1973). However, she failed to ask searching questions regarding the motivations of nurses or their relationships with doctors, hospital managers, patients or society at large. Similarly, despite discussing other occupations open to women in the second half of the nineteenth century (shop assistant, teacher and office worker among them), Holcombe made no comparisons between them. Nevertheless, her work is still widely quoted when the rise of modern nursing is discussed, indicating the scarcity of studies on the subject.

These several works were in the minority, and the history of nursing continues to be largely ignored by other academic disciplines, to this day. While new approaches to nursing history have begun to emerge, the old style, personality-focused work continues.[8]

Celia Davies, Christopher Maggs and Anne Summers have, however, encouraged the emergence of a more academically rigorous approach to nursing history, written by nurses trained as professional historians.[9]

Throughout the 1990s, and into the twenty-first century, the discipline of nursing history in England has shown signs of flourishing, albeit at a slower pace than Maggs' predicted 'flood' (Sweet 2007). Perhaps one of the barriers is the paucity of potential publishers, with the closure of the only British journal dedicated to nursing history in 2003, and the continuing low level of interest in nursing history from women's and gender studies.[10]

In one of the most recent collections of essays on nursing history, Barbara Mortimer has criticized this lack of progress, stating that, 'the contribution that nursing history could make to the wider historiography of women is yet to be fully realised' (Mortimer 2005: 5). Her arguments echo those made by American nurse historian, Patricia D'Antonio, six years earlier, who described the 'two way street' between nursing history and other disciplines as having 'seen much of its intellectual traffic slow to a crawl' (1999: 270). Both writers demonstrate their frustration with the slow evolution of nursing history as a tool through which to view the larger questions concerning women's identity and role in society, and these sentiments have been echoed even more recently in Helen Sweet's exploration of nursing history's historiography (2007).

In a satisfying symmetry, Celia Davies entered the debate once more. In 2007, she reprised the progress made since her initial call to action in 1980, in an article entitled 'Rewriting the History of Nursing – Again?' Her most telling conclusion, after nearly 30 years of endeavour, was 'nursing historians and historians of nursing [are] not only carrying out historical scholarship but also still, to an important extent, fighting to establish the conditions under which that scholarship is possible' (Davies 2007: 25).

Nursing history has progressed from hagiographic and heroic accounts to a more analytical approach. There has been a shift away from the progressive discourses which attempted to plot nursing's inevitable rise from mid-nineteenth-century chaos to the professionalism of the late twentieth century, towards more focused studies of defined topics in closely bounded time periods. Most researchers now incorporate critical appraisal of contemporary material in their work, balancing discussion of content with motive. Contextualization of developments in nursing (within the framework of women's, gender and labour studies) is also growing, although contributions from researchers from within these disciplines is still sparse.

American nurse historian, Joan Lynaugh, has recently identified eight areas of nursing history which should be the focus of future research: among these are nursing knowledge, religious influences and the impact of gender (Lynaugh 2005). To her list could be added the impact of nineteenth-century reforms on the lives and work of ordinary nurses (which will be addressed in this book), nursing in the interwar period and beyond, and the development of specialist branches of nursing, such as children's nursing and asylum nursing.

Christopher Maggs' appeal for more local studies in nursing history has not proved so productive, and few have taken up this particular challenge. The nature of the work makes it time consuming, especially for nurse historians who are required to accommodate their historical research within a larger framework of nursing responsibilities. However, recent advances in online access to census records and other official documents have rendered this type of research more feasible, and large local studies, of the type presented here, will in time emerge. At least one is currently in progress: a study of nineteenth-century private nurse institutions, which aims to track the development of the organizations and the careers of the women who worked in them.

Methodology and sources

This book sets out to address some of the questions raised above. Although it centres on one London teaching hospital, St George's, the findings are discussed in relation to practices at other hospitals. It addresses, directly, Maggs' call for detailed local studies of the lives of ordinary nurses. The time period, from 1850 to 1900, covers an era of great change in nursing in Britain, enabling the impact of reforms to be investigated. St George's was chosen as the case study because of its rich and underused archive, and the discussions therefore necessarily centre on the development of nursing in voluntary general hospitals. Other forms of nursing, such as private and district nursing, are referred to for purposes of comparison.

The dual purposes of the study – to reveal the changing nature of nursing over time and to develop an understanding of the women who chose to work as nurses – required a new approach to research. The paucity (or complete absence) of direct evidence, in the form of diaries, letters or notebooks, constituted a major barrier to the project. Instead, a prosopographical approach was adopted to construct a database of nurses at St George's Hospital between 1850 and 1900 which could be used to study the social mobility and composition of its community of nurses.[11] By using this approach, not only could the changing social structure of the nursing department be revealed, but the lives of nurses who worked at the hospital could also be reconstructed.[12] Six such lives have been selected for publication. They are dispersed throughout the book in the form of pen portraits, in some way compensating for an almost complete lack of visual record of the nurses of St George's.

The archives of St George's Hospital form the heart of the study. The records are rich, and include Nurse Registers, wage books and the minutes of the Weekly Management Board and the Committee for Nursing. These provided insight into the nurses' lives at the hospital, but said little about them before or after their service. A variety of non-hospital sources was consulted to address these gaps, chief among which were the British census returns for the period 1841 to 1901.[13] These were used to locate women both before and after they joined St George's, providing information on family background and subsequent career. Nursing journals were also scanned to find appointments, promotions and other information which could be used to build a picture of women's lives.

The Hospital and the *Nursing Record* provide excellent coverage of the late nineteenth-century debates which split nursing asunder. Both had colourful editors who took opposing sides in the registration debate, and it is important to understand their politics when using these sources. *The Hospital* (first published in 1886) was against registration, and was the official organ of Henry Burdett's Hospital Association. The *Nursing Record* (first published in 1888 and decidedly pro-registration) was edited first by Charles Rideal and then by Ethel Fenwick. It was closely associated with the British Nurses' Association (RBNA). In April 1888, in response to the launch of the *Nursing Record*, *The Hospital* introduced a special supplement, the *Nursing Mirror*, while the *Nursing Record* extended its title to the *Nursing Record and Hospital World*, in October 1893, to widen its brief to include hospital business in general.

Finally, Charles Booth's highly informative, yet woefully underused, survey of matrons from a number of London hospitals, conducted in the mid-1890s, provides unusual insight into the thoughts of leading matrons in London at the time on the structure and nature of nursing at their hospitals.[14]

1   The search for self-esteem

Developments in nursing in the late nineteenth century took place against a backdrop of social and scientific upheaval, and it is impossible to frame a discussion of 'new nursing' without placing it in this context. This first chapter will examine two themes which have particular relevance to the subject – the organization of healthcare provision in Victorian England and the changing role of women in Victorian society. Both made a significant contribution to the rise in respectability of nursing, which occurred in the second half of the century, and which, in turn, led to the emergence of the 'modern nurse'.

Healthcare and the Victorians

Nineteenth-century healthcare in England resembled a complex web of institutions and practitioners (Rivett 1986). Most sick people were cared for at home, regardless of social background, and unlike today, hospitals were almost exclusively the domain of the poor. Among higher social classes, it was almost unheard of to venture inside a hospital as a patient (Woodward 1974; Summers 1989). In fact, the voluntary hospitals had a very narrow remit, focusing on certain classes of disease and a specific section of society. Chronic or 'incurable' cases were only reluctantly admitted, and admission was usually refused to those with infectious fevers; paupers were not welcome. Such patients were increasingly catered for in state-run institutions, such as the fever hospitals and workhouse infirmaries, which burgeoned in the second half of the nineteenth century (Crowther 1981; Ayers 1971).

   In mid-century, workhouse infirmaries were little more than dormitories attached to the main workhouse building, where the sick were nursed by able-bodied female inmates. Louisa Twining, among others, led an outcry against conditions in the workhouses which resulted in a gradual improvement in both accommodation and quality of nursing. As the existing wards became increasingly overcrowded – populated by incurables, the elderly and the chronically sick – separate buildings began to appear, constructed specifically for their treatment (Crowther 1981; Kirby 2002). At the same time trained nurses were gradually introduced (Ayers 1971).

The voluntary hospitals and workhouse infirmaries could not be described as constituting a continuum within a system of healthcare, but operated in relative independence of each other. It was the emergence of Poor Law fever hospitals in London, under the auspices of the Metropolitan Asylums Board (MAB), which heralded the first centrally planned service. In the 1870s, five such hospitals were established in outlying areas of the capital, and all cases of notifiable infectious fevers, whether originating in Poor Law institutions, voluntary hospitals or elsewhere, were supposed to be sent to the new MAB hospitals (Rivett 1986; Ayers 1971).

Victorian asylums for the insane also formed a branch of the state sector, under the auspices of the Poor Law. Such institutions burgeoned in number and size from the 1830s on, as inmates with mental health problems transferred from overcrowded workhouses to relieve pressure on their accommodation. Unlike other institutions, the asylums employed large numbers of male nurses (Jones 1972; Carpenter 1980; Wright 1996).

Patients who could not, or would not, enter an institution had access to a range of alternatives, choice being dictated by their financial situation. Much of the burden for caring for the sick was carried by immediate family or neighbours, but even the poor could sometimes afford a domiciliary nurse (Summers 1989; Rafferty 1995; Wildman 2006). For those with the money, doctors and surgeons were always on hand to visit and treat patients in their own homes. The early domiciliary nurses were a heterogeneous and independent group of self-trained women, often employed by doctors, but who also worked on their own account (Summers 1989). With the emergence of nursing sisterhoods in mid-century this branch of nursing gradually became more formalized, and developed into two strands: private nurses for those who could pay and the forerunners of district nurses for those who could not. William Rathbone's Liverpool Nursing Institution spawned a host of regional institutions for the sick poor in the 1860s, while a similar organization in London (headed by Frances Lees) evolved into the nationwide Queen Victoria Jubilee Institute for Nurses (Damant 2005; Sweet and Dougal 2008; Wildman 2006, 2009). Private nursing institutions did not necessarily restrict their activities to nursing either the poor or the better off. In fact, many used income generated by fee-paying clients to subsidize their work with those less fortunate.

Even within the voluntary sector there was growing diversification. Large teaching hospitals in metropolitan centres were complemented by cottage hospitals in urban and rural settings, and a breathtaking array of specialist hospitals emerged to treat all manner of conditions, such as St Mark's Hospital for the Treatment of Fistula and The Oxygen Home 'for the treatment of ulcers and wounds by Oxygen Gas' (Granshaw 1981; Burdett 1900).

The growth of voluntary hospitals and home visiting institutions provides evidence of the philanthropic nature of Victorian society. From the smallest specialist to the largest teaching hospital, they relied upon public subscriptions and donations for survival (Rivett 1986).[1] While healthcare for the pauper classes was funded through the civic purse, the deserving poor relied on the goodwill and philanthropic ardour of their fellow man (Waddington 2000).

The voluntary hospitals (which form the focus of this book) were, therefore, just one element in a complex Victorian medical marketplace. They were important employers of nurses but were not the only option for women who chose nursing as a career. However, as we will see, they did become a primary locus of training, and by the end of the century, the majority of trained nurses would have passed through a voluntary hospital.

The changing role of women in Victorian society

The development of nursing during the Victorian period can only be fully understood in the context of wider societal changes, and in particular, the changing role of women in nineteenth-century England. The relocation of the nurse from the domestic setting into the hospital, nursing's relationship with the medical profession, the schisms within the nursing profession and its supposed gentrification, must be situated alongside work in gender and women's history.

The role of middle-class women in nineteenth-century society has been the subject of many conflicting narratives in the last 20 years, and can no longer be explained simply in terms of subordination to patriarchal dominance (Gleadle 2001). Recent scholarship, 'led by feminist revival ... combined with the growth of social history and the left-wing desire to recapture "history from below" ', has generated new perspectives (Gleadle 2001: 1).

The traditional view of a typical Victorian middle-class woman was summarized by Amanda Vickery:

> A prisoner in the home, Mrs Average led a sheltered life drained of economic purpose and public responsibility. As her physicality was cramped by custom, corset and crinoline, she was ... a delicate creature ... conspicuously in need of masculine protection ... prey to invalidism. And yet she abjured self-indulgence, being ever-attentive and subservient to the needs of her family. ... She was immured in the private sphere and would not escape till feminism released her.
>
> (A. Vickery 1998: 297)

Vickery's portrait deliberately verges on caricature, but nevertheless, alludes to elements of Victorian society which are hard to refute. Most middle-class Victorian women did not work; their main focus was home and family; and they were outwardly influenced by Christian values. Their lives were governed by the ideology of domesticity; but traditional and feminist historians fervently disagree on the impact such ideology and its associated theoretical constraints had on Victorian women (A. Vickery 1998). While traditional historians continue to portray them as subservient creatures dominated by a patriarchal society, feminists – such as Gamarnikow and Vickery – argue that, far from submitting to the ideology, middle-class Victorian women used it to construct their own place in the public sphere (Gamarnikow 1991; A. Vickery 1998).

Several ideologies conspired to restrict Victorian middle-class women to their homes: Evangelicalism, the ideology of domesticity, and the concept of a society divided into two spheres (public and private) all played their part (Hall 1979; A. Vickery 1998; Summers 2000; Gleadle 2001; Davidoff and Hall 2002).

The rise of Evangelicalism in the early nineteenth century had a significant influence on the role of women. A highly influential (and principally Anglican) movement, which reflected many beliefs of earlier puritan Protestants, it had come to prominence at the end of the previous century, and continued to be dominant through the first half of the nineteenth. Evangelicals had two primary goals: to end the slave trade and to reform the nation's morals and manners – endangered by the supposed collapse of civilized society (Davidoff and Hall 2002). Political and social unrest following the French Revolution, and the gathering pace of industrialization presaged a disintegration of civilization, it was feared (Boyd 1991; Thompson 1988; Best 1979). The agricultural and industrial revolutions, which caused massive relocation of people from the countryside to the cities, added to the ferment; out of which grew a form of paranoia among the upper classes, convinced that working men were on the brink of revolution (Cannadine 1998).

Evangelicals saw it as their duty to steer society back to stability. Led by an influential group of mercantile and landed gentry – known as the Clapham Sect – they used political influence rather than the pulpit to solicit support. Their first targets were the aristocracy and upper classes of society, and then focus switched to the emerging middle classes (Hall 1979). The political interests of the middle classes and the Evangelical movement were mutually supportive. While the middle classes provided a large and growing base for support of Evangelical reform, Evangelicalism's political connections offered opportunities to take advantage of the newly extended franchise (Hall 1979; Cannadine 1998). Additionally, Evangelical morality, centred firmly on home and family, was seen as an effective antidote to the moral dangers of industrial capitalism. It transformed the home from a mere 'place of peaceful refuge' (as it had been portrayed the century before) into 'a sacred place, a quasi-religious centre to men's lives … and bulwark against … political subversion' (Trudgill 1976: 39–41). The 'Evangelical home' offered a safe haven from the unparalleled pace of change afflicting Victorian society. The importance of Evangelicalism in defining Victorian society cannot be overstated; as Catherine Hall, has written, it 'was probably the single most widespread influence in Victorian England' (Hall 1979: 15).

The Evangelical ideology of domesticity had a profound effect on the role of women, especially when combined with early Victorian interpretations of natural differences between the sexes. Women were defined by their biological function to bear and raise children, and this alone would have been sufficient to confine them to the home. Their moral strength was questioned: they were weak in the face of temptation – an opinion which can be traced to belief in Original Sin – and driven by their emotions, unable to 'disentangle their passions from their reasoning'. Adding physical weakness to the list, women were ill-equipped to face the dangers of the outside world (Burstyn 1980: 72). As a result they were 'a source of constant anxiety to men [and] only with outside help from religion and from men who cared for them could women develop self control' (Burstyn 1980: 72). In many respects, they were regarded by their menfolk as little more than 'children of a larger growth', their whims and fancies tolerated, as children's were, but never taken seriously (Trudgill 1976: 67).[2]

This infantilization of women was reinforced through law. Until the Married Women's Property Act of 1873, women had few rights, and even the children of a marriage were considered to be the property of the father. The introduction of the 1873 Act marked an irreversible decline in the autocratic authority wielded by husbands over their wives; but unmarried daughters remained tightly supervised, confined within the protective boundaries of the family (Harris 1993).

The Victorian view of women as weak innocents, in need of protection from corrupting forces, lies at the root of this protective relationship (Davidoff 1983). Complex chaperoning arrangements and close surveillance of daughters were essential for the protection of this innocence, loss of which rebounded not just on the unfortunate daughter, but on her whole family (Cominos 1980). The home was the natural place for women. Here, they could be protected from the ravages of the outside world and make best use of their inherent attributes, as wives and mothers. Paradoxically, within the home, women's weaknesses became strengths – reinterpreted as nurture, empathy and morality – which could be mustered to protect the family against dissolute outside influences (Hall 1979). Predisposed to religion, by dint of purity and lack of exposure to moral dangers, women were regarded as the natural keepers of the family's moral health and religious sensibilities (Hall 1979). Further, safe within the family, women acquired a wisdom and strength which was wholly missing from their 'outdoor' personas. As domestic ideology acquired importance in the fight against societal breakdown, women's role as guardians of the ideology transformed them into proselytizers of middle-class morals and manners among the lower classes (Trudgill 1976).

Despite this central role in family life, women maintained a subordinate and deferential position to their husbands. Family structure mirrored that of society, which, according to Leonora Davidoff, was represented as an organic body of, 'hierarchically ordered but interdependent parts' (1983: 19). The Head (the 'thinking organ' or the brain) was represented in society by governing upper- or middle-class males, and in the family by the husband. The Hands (the 'unthinking and unfeeling doers') were society's working classes, and servants in the domestic economy. Middle-class wives were the 'Heart of the family, its Soul, the seat of tenderness, morality and the emotions' (Davidoff 1983: 19). The analogy of women as the family's heart and soul becomes important when considering the roles they were permitted to assume in the outside world.

The second defining ideology of the Victorian period, that of the 'two spheres', worked with domesticity to further restrict middle-class women's movements. It followed logically from the Evangelicals' world view. Outside the home – the public sphere – was danger, both moral and physical. It was the domain of men. Inside the home – the private sphere – was woman's domain. Here, her natural, nurturing talents held sway (Hall 1979).

By the mid-nineteenth century, these two ideologies had become tightly woven into the fabric of middle-class life, and as the century progressed, despite a decline in the number of seriously religious, they had become synonymous with this section of society (Best 1985; Davidoff and Hall 2002). Although the old threats to society had receded, new ones emerged. Technological advances in transport and communication generated an almost frightening pace of life, and the home continued to represent a safe place of refuge from the outside world (Trudgill 1976).

From the 1870s, as the doctrine came under challenge from the nascent feminist movement, advances in scientific thinking were pressed into its support. A new understanding of reproductive biology enabled doctors to claim that women were in thrall to the 'involuntary periodicity of their reproductive systems'; while Social Darwinists used evolutionary theory to 'prove' that women (like children, the working classes and native inhabitants of colonial lands) were naturally inferior to their menfolk (Poovey 1989; Davidoff 1983; Burstyn 1980; McDermid 1995; Vicinus 1985). Both arguments were used with great force to shore up the barriers which kept middle-class women from participating in the public sphere, which, by this time, were in danger of being breached.

The ideology was appropriated to promote specific causes. Trade unions used it to great effect to exclude women, accused of taking jobs from their better paid male colleagues, from the workplace. If women's natural place was in the home, they argued, it followed that their presence in the workplace was unnatural (Rose 1992).

The domesticity/separate spheres construct was closely associated with yet another Victorian obsession, respectability; a combination which added further pressure on women to remain indoors. Respectability was an aspiration which permeated Victorian life across the classes (Best 1985; Thompson 1988). It was possible to be respectable and working-class, just as it was possible to be a member of the upper classes yet not respectable (Best 1985; Cordery 1995). Measures of respectability differed between the sexes, and were closely linked to gender attributes: male respectability entailed being strong, brave and independent; for women, it required sexual purity, domesticity and motherhood (Rose 1992). The most important attribute for men was independence, and the obligation to provide for the family was paramount. In a world of increasingly conspicuous consumerism, fuelled by the growth in capitalist industrialization, a leisured wife and a staff of servants became very public signs of a man's respectability and success. For middle-class women, this aspect of respectability became a major obstacle to venturing out of the family home, especially to undertake paid employment.[3] A 'working lady' was a contradiction in terms: a wife who worked brought shame on her husband, implying he was incapable of supporting his family through his own labours (Holcombe 1973: 4).

The triumvirate of domesticity, two spheres and respectability therefore conspired to confine the Victorian middle-class woman to the home; and yet, in apparent contradiction, she was expected to venture into the most dangerous of places to undertake work with the poor. It was her key duty to society, to reform the morals and manners (and therefore control the behaviour) of the lower classes. With her education in religion and domestic management, and inherent female attributes of empathy, tenderness and purity, the middle-class woman was admirably equipped for the work (Prochaska 1980). Her religiosity obliged her to undertake such duties, despite the dangers to her own moral well-being. As Hannah More, a leading member of the Clapham Sect, said '[It] is the calling of a lady; the care of the poor is her profession' (quoted in Hall 1979: 28).

Upper- and middle-class anxieties with regard to their social inferiors – and the desire to control them – were compounded by an increasing physical separation, as the middle classes moved out to suburban locations (Dyhouse 1976). Visiting the poor became an essential means of maintaining contact with this morally suspect group, providing reminders of the values of respectable society which had otherwise become physically remote (Summers 1979). One social commentator, in 1844, said of the Manchester social elite that they 'knew no more of the working classes than they did of the inhabitants of New Zealand or Kamchatka' (quoted in Cannadine 1998: 83).[4] The Reverend J.S. Brewster, in 1855, urged ladies to visit the inmates of workhouses, with a similar warning, 'If you do not know what they do, neither do they know what you do' (quoted in Summers 1979: 40). Both argued that the most effective way to influence the lower classes was to infiltrate their homes, and thereby, their minds and manners.

There were practical reasons which made middle-class women ideal candidates for this work, as well as ideological arguments: they had already had direct contact with the working classes through their management of domestic servants (Summers 1979). As men withdrew from contact with their lower-class employees, women's contact was extending across the class barriers. The inter-class relationships within the home (between mistress and servants) became a model for similar relationships outside it. Summers quotes Brewster again, to illustrate the point:

> [Those] you have ... instructed in their respective duties – whose manners you have softened – who have learnt from you how to manage a household – who have caught from you, insensibly, lessons of vast utility ... order ... economy ... cleanliness ... management of children, of household comfort and tidiness...
>
> (quoted in Summers 1979: 40)

This was the objective of visitation, to take middle-class values and inculcate them into the homes of the poor; and as guardians of those values, women were best placed to undertake the task. Summers has further argued that the middle-class woman gained practical benefit from such contact: it brought her into contact with potential recruits to her household, and provided opportunities to train them for domestic work, before they were actually employed (Summers 1979).

Women's philanthropic work outside the home was therefore perceived as an extension of their work within it, and in this way barriers to women undertaking roles in the 'public' sphere were lowered, to a limited extent. The Victorian emphasis on 'citizenship of contribution' supported this role for women in the public domain, their work with the poor being conceptualized as their 'moral contribution' to society (Digby and Stewart 1996; Gleadle 2001). They were transferring their role as the 'heart and soul' of the family into the wider sphere; and as most women worked with their local poor, it could be viewed more as an extended private sphere than a move into the male-dominated public sphere proper (Digby and Stewart 1996). Women thus constructed a 'borderland' between public and private spheres, enabling them to move out of the home, into a public space which was predominantly theirs (Digby 1992). Their activities in this small public space were severely limited, and still ultimately controlled by men who managed the philanthropic organizations, such as the Visiting Societies, through which they worked (Prochaska 1980). While respectable women might undertake nurturing roles in society, their respectability would immediately be questioned if there was any hint of involvement in commerce, as managing even a philanthropic organization might suggest.

Middle-class women's philanthropic activity burgeoned. After the Poor Law Act of 1834, a new form of visitation gradually emerged, as women began to include public institutions in their rounds. Curtailment of outdoor relief forced the poor into workhouses in increasing numbers and the locus of lady visitors' work shifted (Summers 1979). This shift took place over several decades, and was fraught with opposition from male managers of these institutions (King 2006). The Workhouse Visiting

Society was founded by Louisa Twining in 1858, but it was only after the 1868 Poor Law Amendment Act, and the fragmentation of the Poor Law system, that women began to gain a real foothold in public institutions (Abel-Smith 1964; Summers 1979). The first female Poor Law guardian was not appointed until 1875 (King 2006).[5] Historians have disagreed over the interpretation of these events. Some argue that early female guardians made little impact on welfare provision, and that many were staunch supporters of the 1834 Poor Law Act, alienating paupers and workhouse staff in equal measure (Crowther 1981; Hollis 1987). A counter-argument claims that such women were able to effect a considerable range of improvements in the treatment of paupers (Summers 1979; Levine 1990; Harris 1993). Whichever interpretation reflects reality, it is clear that the Workhouse Visiting Society marked an important milestone in the professionalization of female philanthropy; a move which, according to Kathryn Gleadle, presaged 'the prominent role women were to play in local government' several decades later (2001: 68).

Ladies also became visitors to hospitals, but failed to achieve the same status. Few hospitals admitted women to the board of management, despite campaigns run by activists arguing for women's involvement in other public institutions. Henrietta Barnett (one of the first female Poor Law guardians to be appointed) promoted the cause of women managers in hospitals, emphasizing their superior qualifications compared to men – as a consequence of their natural abilities in caring for the sick (Waddington 2003). Hospitals resisted. With the exception of a few specialist institutions, women continued to be excluded from hospital boards to the end of the century.[6] Even where they were tolerated, their sphere of influence was restricted to areas deemed most appropriate – such as the management of the matron or the wards. They were rarely (if ever) empowered to influence the financial management of the institution.[7] The complexity of voluntary hospitals, and their finances, resembled business (entrenching them within the public, or male, sphere); it was a step too far to permit women to become involved in their management (Waddington 2003).

Lady visitors faced great obstacles in most public institutions. Permission to visit was obtained from male managers who were often of a lower social class, and harboured much suspicion of their motives. These unwanted 'guests' were regarded as a, 'meddling interference, busy bodies which [*sic*] might expose abuses' (Prochaska 1980: 141). Managers accused women of moving out of their own sphere, and encroaching on the public realm, but this disapproval was probably based as much on class differences as on discourses concerned with gender (Summers 1979).

Supporters of women's involvement in the public sphere turned the tables on their opponents, using the same rhetoric of domesticity to facilitate their introduction into public institutions. Women had natural skills completely lacking in male managers: 'There was little in [their] training which prepared them for the internal management of an orphanage or a home for widows. Nor did they speak the same language of the matrons and nurses who staffed their institutions' (Prochaska 1980: 143). Women, on the other hand, learnt these skills at their mothers' side. They should be the mistresses of institutions, as the male heads were the masters. As Catherine Cappe (a Unitarian philanthropist who campaigned for women visitors in public and charitable institutions) explained,

> A lady visitor in an Hospital or Asylum, should be to that institution what the kind judicious Mistress of a family is to her household – the careful inspector of the economy, the integrity and the good moral conduct of the housekeeper and other inferior servants.
>
> (Quoted in Prochaska 1980: 141)

Florence Nightingale used similar imagery to rationalize the presence of lady nurses in hospital wards, equating the relationship between nurse and patient (of any age) to that of mother and child. Her advice to new nurses emphasized this, 'while you have a ward it must be your *home*, and its inmates must be your children' (Prochaska 1980: 147).[8]

By the mid-nineteenth century, for some single middle-class women, philanthropic work, had become more than simply an obligation. It developed into a way of life, or an occupation (albeit unpaid), which enabled them to combine religious duty with a fulfilling role (Prochaska 1980). Frustrated by their restrictive home-life (and lack of access to the education received by their brothers) intelligent, middle-class women, seized on philanthropic work as an outlet (Deane 1996). Louisa Twining dedicated her life to philanthropic work, gradually extending her influence well beyond her immediate locality to become involved in national issues including the election of women to Poor Law boards and reform of the workhouse system (Deane 1996). According to Deane, the motivation for women like Twining was not religious duty alone, but encompassed a 'search for self-esteem and self-actualisation' (Deane 1996: 138).

A literal interpretation of the two-spheres ideology has led twentieth-century historians to construct the traditional image of middle-class Victorian women as subdued, oppressed, passive beings. Feminist historians have questioned the orthodoxy of separate spheres, arguing that there are contradictions within it which are difficult to resolve. On the one hand women were regarded as the moral guardians of their families, but at the same time were considered morally weak (Digby 1992). Similarly, women were constrained to the home, but were obliged (by a mix of civic and religious duty) to work with the poor in their own world. Amanda Vickery has suggested that the separate spheres construct was primarily a rhetorical device, used to counter a perceived increase in the public presence of women (1998). Further, she claims that the contradictions were used by women to great effect, to create spaces within the public sphere which they could occupy (A. Vickery 1998). Far from being subordinated, Vickery argues, detailed studies of individuals and groups reveal Victorian women to be 'spirited, capable and, most importantly, diverse' (A. Vickery 1998: 300).

The rise in respectability of nursing and the emergence of the new nurse

Vickery's arguments underline the importance of questioning received notions of Victorian society and similar questions can be asked of Victorian nursing.

Historians cannot agree on the origins of the 'revolution in nursing', as Dingwall *et al.* have described it, although most now concur that the basis for modern nursing in England lay in the work of the sisterhoods, and in particular the work of Elizabeth Fry, in the early 1840s (Dingwall *et al.* 1988). There is also a consensus that, by the end of the century, nursing was accepted as a suitable occupation for single middle-class women, although debates persist as to the extent to which it had become dominated by such women, as this study will demonstrate.

How nursing attained this status, and how middle-class women were persuaded to join in great numbers is also the subject of continuing debate. Nursing in the second half of the nineteenth century, on first sight, would seem eminently unsuitable for respectable women. Every aspect threatened 'loss or absence of caste' (Summers 2000: 87). It required women to move away from the safety of home into the public sphere; the work was of a manual nature, involved taking rather than giving orders, and brought them into daily, intimate contact with non-family members of the opposite sex, both doctors and patients (Summers 2000). Male working-class patients, particularly, presented a serious moral and spiritual danger. Later in the century, years after middle-class women's space in hospitals had been successfully negotiated, other employers were still inventing ways to protect the modesty of their newly found middle-class female workforce, by physically dividing the workplace along gender lines. Lady clerks at the Prudential Insurance Company, for example, were accommodated in separate offices, had their own relaxation areas and even their own staircases, so there was no danger of inadvertent contact with male colleagues (Jordan 1996; Davin 2005).

Concern for the moral and spiritual health of working women even extended to working-class women in factories. Reformers of factory legislation focused on the potential dangers to the moral health of factory women (and therefore their families) of mingled sexes in the workplace, rather than the dangers of unsafe machinery or excessively long hours of work (Alexander 1976).

In hospitals, separation of the sexes was impossible. Instead, the presence of middle-class nurses was justified as an extension of philanthropic visitation; and ladies' committees were used as a precedent for their acceptance. By extending the boundaries of the private sphere, middle-class women could assume the mantle of 'mother' to the hospital's patients, infantilizing the inmates and effectively rendering contact between male patient and female nurse non-sexual (Prochaska 1980). Nightingale, who used this image repeatedly, also emphasized the importance of an unblemished character and the need for moral strength. The new nurse was thus constructed in the image of a saint or an angel, untouchable and asexual (Trudgill 1976; Judd 1998).[9] The use of the family metaphor also, conveniently, reinforced existing patriarchal hierarchies which placed doctors (and male managers) in control. Thus the presence of middle-class women in hospitals was naturalized through the construct of domesticity and a space was created for them in what otherwise would have been contentious territory (Gamarnikow 1978). The benefits of this space, once created, were laid clear: in institutions populated by the morally weak (working classes), lady nurses had a captive audience for their Evangelical teachings on morality, economy and efficiency. Attention to patients' physical health could be combined with similar attention to their moral and spiritual well-being. Other employees in the hospital were also expected to benefit from this influence.

The 1856 takeover of nursing at King's College Hospital by the St John's House Sisterhood was one of the first examples of middle-class nurses moving into hospitals (Moore 1988).[10] Since the Reformation, the close association between religious practitioners and the care of the sick had been dissolved. But, prompted by the growth in religiosity in the early nineteenth century, groups of middle- and upper-class women joined together to form loose congregations with the objective of resurrecting this relationship.[11] The sisterhoods provided women with an opportunity to practise a more organized form of philanthropy and, operating under the auspices of the Church, they were afforded more freedom in their actions (Vicinus 1985). Most recruited their sisters from the middle and upper classes, while their nurses came from lower ranks in society (Moore 1988). It was the task of the sisters to instil middle-class Christian morality and discipline in their working-class subordinates. While the nurses were paid, the sisters usually worked on a voluntary basis – thus sidestepping the proscription on working ladies – and even contributed financially to the running of the institution. Though the sisterhoods were run in accordance with Victorian middle-class sensitivities, the women still had to negotiate their territory very carefully; but through their focus on religious and charitable activities, they were able to push back the boundaries to create their own space within the public sphere (Helmstadter 1996 and 2001; Summers 2000). It should be no surprise, then, that nursing sisterhoods provided the first middle-class nurses to hospitals. With their strong sense of Christian morality they were deemed to be as safe as it was possible to be from the corrupting influence of public hospitals.

These roots of nursing, in the mid-century sisterhoods, lie at the heart of its characterization as a vocation rather than a mere occupation. Anne Summers has claimed that it was precisely this vocational element which enabled respectable women to enter such a sordid occupation, an argument also used by Likeman, in her discussion of nursing at the end of the century (Summers 2000; Likeman 2002). Summers has further argued that nursing reforms arose out of a perception that the working poor were in need of spiritual ministry, which reformed nurses were ideally placed to provide (1991). Others have argued that vocation was nothing more than a convenient cloak used by nurse reformers to maintain respectability. It also helped to obviate any potential threat to doctors, which the presence of middle-class women in hospitals might otherwise pose (Helmstadter 2003). The requirement for outward respectability dominated women's employment throughout the century, whether in hospitals, local government, on school boards, or as teachers. All women thus employed were obliged to '[Cloak] themselves, to a quite exaggerated degree, with modesty, propriety and other outward trappings of femininity' (Harris 1993: 26). Only in this way could they protect their reputations, maintain respectability and reduce the threat they posed to the natural order.

However, nursing sisterhoods were viewed with increasing suspicion by hospital governors, tainted by their perceived association with attempts to romanize the Church of England. Although instrumental in the early days of nursing reform, their influence waned as the century progressed (Poovey 1989). Only three of the large London hospitals entrusted their nursing departments to the hands of a sisterhood: King's College and Charing Cross were nursed at various times by St John's House, while the All Saints Sisterhood nursed UCH.[12]

The trappings of religion were not entirely abandoned by nursing, and it continued to be represented (by Nightingale and other reformers) as a Christian vocation, entailing self-sacrifice, devotion and moral certainty. These characteristics also defined middle-class womanhood (the good mother, obedient wife and daughter and moral core of the family) making nursing less alien to such women. Nightingale's mantra, that a good nurse was also a good woman, reinforced these connections (Rafferty 1996; Bradshaw 2000). Women were natural nurses, according to Nightingale and other reformers, and required training only in the efficient employment of those skills to the benefit of the patient (Versluysen 1980; Simonton 2001).[13]

The focus on the character of nurses served several purposes. As reformers of working-class morals, it ensured they were the 'embodiment of Christian virtue' necessary for their work as reformers of working-class morals (Rafferty 1996: 13). It also ensured that they were well equipped to withstand challenges to their own moral health posed by exposure to dangerous influences encountered in the hospitals. The characteristics which constituted a good nurse were repeated endlessly, generating an image of nursing familiar to middle-class women, and reinforcing the impression that it was a respectable profession. As Alison Bashford has argued, 'ordering, cleansing, purifying and moralising ... had come to be so firmly the territory of the middle-class women' that the role of nurse became synonymous with them, and their presence became a necessity for the modernization of hospitals (Bashford 1998: xv). The primacy of character training over any other elements of nurse education would become a contended space in the vigorous debates on nurse registration later in the century.

The presence of lady visitors who dispensed kind words and spiritual guidance throughout the wards of voluntary hospitals, no doubt eased the way for lady nurses. At St George's, lady visitors were assigned to specific wards and visited on a weekly basis (SGHWB/31 30 November 1859). Although occasionally involved in investigations into complaints, they had no apparent direct influence on the hospital's management. At other hospitals, they played a more active role. Lady visitors to the Hospital for Sick Children at Great Ormond Street (HSC) appeared to have more influence, although they were never elected to either the Management Committee or the Board of Governors. A committee of such women (comprising, among others, Louisa Twining and the wives of several eminent doctors) reported on the state of nursing in the hospital in 1860. Most of its recommendations were ignored – much to Louisa Twining's disgust – but their main recommendation, to replace the old Matron with a Lady Superintendent, was implemented (GOS5/2/30, November 1860). The arrival of a 'lady' superintendent opened the doors to a stream of well-bred young women, appointed as sisters on a voluntary basis.

It was important for nurse reformers to represent hospitals as safe places, where a middle-class woman's reputation and respectability would be protected; and this importance grew as the century progressed and recruits became younger. The need for parental approval became paramount. As a result, in addition to emphasizing the moral qualities of nursing, a heavy emphasis was placed on discipline and supervision. At the Nightingale School, special measures were introduced to protect the reputations of probationers. They worked on self-contained wards, minimizing the need to move around the hospital; and wards were structured such that probationers (and patients) were under the gaze of authority. Access to the outside world was circumscribed to protect the young women from the insalubrious surroundings of the hospital (Rafferty 1996). Much of this discipline was designed to reassure parents, 'often horrified at the notion of their daughters working in centres of sin and sickness', as hospitals were generally regarded (Vicinus 1985: 87).[14] As Rafferty commented, 'The nurses' home provided the necessary level of moral tutelage to assuage the fears of anxious parents allowing their daughters to live away from home' (1996: 35).

This focus on discipline and morality was not restricted to nursing. Discipline, essential for the maintenance of respectability, was the cornerstone for all new communities of women which arose in the second half of the nineteenth century (Vicinus 1985). In hospitals, though, discipline reached new heights. Strict codes of conduct and a complex etiquette for managing relationships evolved to a much higher degree than in most other organizations which opened their doors to women (Vicinus 1985). Unlike women's colleges or non-nursing sisterhoods (or even the Prudential) it was not feasible to maintain complete separation of male and female workers, while interaction with male patients (sometimes of a very intimate nature) was a routine part of the job. Contact was heavily regulated and obedience demanded. A probationer at the Nightingale School described how relations between doctors and nurses were supposed to be conducted: 'We are not supposed to have anything to say to [medical students] except in connection with the work', she wrote to a friend (quoted in Vicinus 1985: 99). But she also commented that it was impossible not to engage in conversation when working closely together, demonstrating the difficulties in maintaining a strict aura of respectability about the wards.

In the Victorian imagination an innocent conversation could easily deteriorate into something far more dangerous if concentration was allowed to lapse. St George's had a complex set of rules governing communication between doctors and nurses, designed to avoid such lapses. Resident Medical Officers were prohibited from talking directly to nurses, even on the topic of patient care. Instead instructions had to be transmitted through the day or night superintendents, who were older women, and presumably less susceptible to moral degeneracy. However, as at St Thomas', it seems that theory and practice may not have coincided, as *The Lancet* referred to this rule as a 'fiction' (*The Lancet*, 18 November 1871: 929).

Middle-class nurses found support among several sections of society. Private clients, with their increasing wealth, sophistication and demand for better quality nursing in the home, welcomed the arrival of middle-class nurses (Williams 1980). Philanthropists and religious groups, recognizing the opportunities they presented for reform of the working classes in hospital wards and in their homes, and also supported the move (Williams 1980). Hospital managers welcomed them more cautiously, believing their respectability would raise the tone of their establishments and facilitate fund-raising. Their skill and experience in managing domestic servants were expected to bring a new discipline to nursing departments, staffed in the main by untrained, working-class women (Rafferty 1996; Bashford 1998). Reservations centred on their potential to disrupt established hospital hierarchies.

Reception by the medical profession was possibly most equivocal, and their reaction can only be understood in the context of fundamental changes taking place in hospitals in the second half of the nineteenth century.[15] Reform of nursing in the mid-century coincided with the beginnings of rapid growth in the hospital system which brought increasing numbers of the sick poor into its domain (Woodward 1974). Between 1861 and 1891, the number of voluntary hospitals in England increased from 153 to 409 and the number of beds from 14,772 to 29,520 (Pinker 1966).

This rapid growth in beds facilitated Victorian obsessions with observing and measuring, and with controlling the working classes, and hospitals offered the opportunity for both reforming the poor and studying and relieving disease (Dean and Bolton 1980). As patients were confined in larger numbers, within special buildings, the science of medicine benefited from this gathering together of so many sick bodies for study (Foucault 1994). But doctors visited their patients infrequently. If details of progress (or otherwise) were to be recorded regularly, they needed a trustworthy aid. It has been suggested that in the new middle-class nurse, doctors found their reliable and trustworthy assistants (Poovey 1989).

Where previously nursing had been a mix of nurturing and manual activities, a need for a new type of nurse, combining skilled observation, attention to detail and some theoretical knowledge, was emerging. One impetus for better trained nurses may then have originated from the doctors, in their need for more skilled partners in the new venture into scientific medicine. Carol Helmstadter claims this contribution has been overshadowed by historians' focus on Nightingale (2002). Other historians have been less generous to the medics, suggesting that the principal attraction of young middle-class nurses lay in their supposed malleability, in comparison to the working-class women with whom they were accustomed to work (Summers 1989; Gamarnikow 1991; Rafferty 1996).

Was it inevitable that nurses should fulfil this new role of skilled technician? Hospital doctors had long been supported by teams of medical clerks and dressers who traditionally undertook most routine tasks. If advances in medicine were generating such work in larger volumes, why were their numbers not simply increased, rather than creating another tribe of medical assistant in the shape of the trained nurse? Professional protectionism may be the explanation (Poovey 1989; Rafferty 1996). Medical clerks and dressers were usually doctors in training; any significant increase in numbers would strain the existing medical monopoly, by creating more qualified doctors than the medical marketplace could support. It also risked widening the 'entry gate' into medicine, at a time when the profession was attempting to tighten access, particularly in respect to the entry of women (Rafferty 1996: 25). Female non-medical attendants (or nurses) were much less of a threat, especially as their leaders were actively promoting reformed nurses as subordinate to the medical profession (Poovey 1989). Using nurses in this new role was safe.

But, although initially greeted with approval, many doctors became wary of the new nurse, fearing the prospect of nurses from a higher social class, possibly closer to the influential governors than they were themselves. The new lady nurses and lady superintendents threatened their autonomy in the hospital, in doctors' eyes at least, and challenged their position at the head of the hierarchy (Vicinus 1985). Nightingale's insistence that nursing should be under the control of 'one female trained head', and that no man (be he a clergyman or doctor) should be permitted to interfere with nursing, cannot have strengthened their fragile egos (quoted in Abel-Smith 1960: 25). Suspicions grew as nurses began to call for more thorough grounding in the medical sciences. The campaign for nurse registration – which began in the late 1880s and was not resolved until 1919 – was the ultimate challenge to medical authority. It incorporated the demand for rigorous scientific education (along the lines of the medical curriculum) with a central nurse-run authority to control entry to the occupation and to define standards. A central system, under the leadership of a senior nurse, removed control from the doctors; the introduction of medical subjects to the nursing curriculum threatened their monopoly over the knowledge base of the profession (Gamarnikow 1991).[16]

Focus on obedience (and use of the family metaphor) was therefore not only important to instil respectability into nursing, but, from the doctors' point of view, critical in maintaining nursing's subordination to the medical profession (Gamarnikow 1978; Versluysen 1980).

The medical profession reverted to gendered arguments based on the dominant role of men, counterpoised against the subservient role of women (Gamarnikow 1991). By repeatedly emphasizing the femininity of nursing, doctors conflated female subordination with nursing's subordination and, by contrast, male power with medical power (Gamarnikow 1991). Surprisingly, this position was also adopted by early nurse leaders, who 'proudly claimed [for nursing] a supportive, subordinate relationship to its male counterpart' (Poovey 1989: 166). According to Mary Poovey, 'this self-proclaimed subordination' was crucial if nursing was to be presented as a respectable occupation. It also neutralized 'the spectre of female sexuality ... associated with independent women' (Poovey 1989: 166). Nightingale and her followers had taken a pragmatic decision: in order to reconstruct nursing as a respectable female occupation – with its own female hierarchy – it must be located firmly within, and subordinate to, the existing medical system.

This approach held sway for two decades, but was challenged in the 1880s by a more radical strategy, typified by Ethel Fenwick and the pro-registrationists. Their goal was to establish nursing as a completely separate profession, independent of the medical faculty. The ensuing bitter debate polarized medical society: both pro- and anti-registrationists could be found in the medical profession, hospital management and nursing itself.

Despite the avowed determination to develop nursing as a profession run by and for nurses, the pro-registrationists lost control of the association founded to promote their cause to a group of medical men and matrons who opposed their views. The Royal British Nurses' Association immediately changed its allegiance and began to lobby against the registration of nurses. It might be asked why an association which aimed to be run by women had invited so many medical men onto its governing bodies?[17] Perhaps, like Nightingale, the pro-registrationists recognized that without the support of members of the medical profession their objectives could not be achieved, but unfortunately, they invited the wrong medical men into their midst. Fenwick and her followers went on to fight the battle through other channels, achieving a central system of registration in 1919.[18]

The decision of both sides to involve medical practitioners in their attempts to carve out a niche for nursing was taken out of pragmatism, but the effects have been felt by successive generations of nurses, as the nursing profession continues to battle for professional parity with doctors.[19]

A combination of medical need, philanthropic fervour and 'rampant snobbery' has been evoked as the underlying cause in the rise of the middle-class nurse, but a more prosaic explanation has also been proposed. It is no coincidence, according to some historians, that the new nurse so closely resembled a middle-class woman; they contend that the role was developed specifically in response to a mid-century demographic and economic crisis, which saw a dramatic rise in the number of unmarried, middle-class women in society.[20]

In 1859, *The Edinburgh Review* published an article by the radical journalist and feminist, Harriet Martineau, on 'redundant women'. Using data from the 1851 census, she highlighted the growing problem of single women, who, with no other means of support, had to rely on their own earnings. Martineau calculated that British women outnumbered men by half a million, and of six million women over the age of 20, more than two million were self-supporting widows or spinsters, with no hope to 'marry and [be] taken care of' (Martineau quoted in Tusan 2000: 221).[21]

Martineau's article focused the public's attention on the plight of single, unsupported women. Identifying suitable occupations for them through which they could support themselves became a clarion call for early feminists. Jessie Boucherett (a member of the Langham Place feminists) set up the Society for Promoting the Employment of Women (SPEW) specifically to help such women find work, often in occupations previously considered inappropriate.[22] The Society acted as employment agency and training centre, providing courses in such diverse skills as book-keeping, law copywriting and printing (Jordan 1999; Tusan 2000).

Single middle-class women were problematic for Victorian society. Working-class women, married or single, had always been expected to contribute to the family income, but for middle-class women, bound by the ideology of domesticity, earning a wage was not an option. The existence of large numbers of unsupported middle-class women threatened the economic stability of society.

William Greg (a social and political commentator of the time) described the unnatural position of such women in no uncertain terms, implying an inherent failure on their part to fulfil the 'natural duties and labour of wives and mothers'. In his words, they were 'abnormal' and 'incomplete' and their occupations were 'artificial' and 'painfully sought' (quoted in Poovey 1989: 1). Single women, with no family or husband to care for, had no place in a society which defined women only in these terms. Furthermore, if forced to undertake paid work to support themselves, they forfeited their respectability, and their station in society fell even further. Many writers warned of the loss of status which attached itself to any respectable woman who took up paid work, as these two quotes illustrate. The first is from 1869, the second from 1881, indicating how entrenched the ideology was.

> A lady may do almost anything from motives of charity or zeal … but [if] a woman begins to receive money, however great her need … the heroine is transformed into a tradeswoman.
> (Mrs Ellis, *Education of the Heart: women's best work*, quoted in Prochaska 1980: 6)

> A lady, to be sure, must be a mere lady and nothing else. She must not work for profit or engage in any occupation that money can command.
> (Mrs E. Genna, *Irresponsible Philanthropists, being some Chapters on the Employment of Gentlewomen*, quoted in Holcombe 1973: 4)

The 'redundant woman problem' was precipitated by the untimely convergence of two social phenomena, already discussed: respectability and the rise of industrialization. The convergence was inevitable as they fed off each other. The rise of capitalist industrialization generated a growing consumerism within the middle classes, and as respectability became increasingly defined by possessions, economic pressure on middle-class families escalated. It became more difficult for fathers to provide for their single daughters. Unable to address the problem by sending them out to work, because of the risk of tarnished respectability, families became trapped in a self-perpetuating dilemma (D'Cruze 2000).

Where did all these single women come from? The origins of the crisis lay in several shifts in the behaviour of the middle classes in the latter part of the nineteenth century. Couples began to marry later in life. The rise in consumerism had forced up the cost of running a respectable household and decisions to marry were postponed, until a couple felt financially able to create a home commensurate with their position in society.[23] Consequently, women stayed single – and dependent – on their fathers or other male relatives for longer periods of time; the years stretching out ahead of them before they could fulfil their natural destiny. The high expectation placed on men to make increasingly extravagant provision for their families led many to choose not to marry at all. They left the country in large numbers, lured by opportunities of the expanding empire (Holcombe 1973).

This explanation creates an image of single middle-class women as a passive creatures, waiting indefinitely under the protection of male relatives for the arrival of a husband. Historians such as Martha Vicinus have argued a different case; that like men, some women decided not to marry. For them, a dearth of marriageable men may have been a boon and spinsterhood offered legitimate escape from the stultifying altern-ative. By remaining single, they could enjoy independent lives, dedicated to many and various causes; social reform, feminism, religion and philan-thropy (Vicinus 1985; A. Vickery 1998).[24] A nurse writing to *The Hospital* substantiates this when she claims that earning her own living generated a 'great joy in the freedom and independence [so gained]'. The restrictive environment of marriage could not compare with the variety and peripa-tetic nature of her work (*H/NM*, 4 August 1888: lxxii). The writer made no allusion to spiritual motivations nor to the warm glow of altruism in knowing one had sacrificed one's life for the sick poor. Her love of nursing was based on the benefits it conferred, among which being free and independent were high on her list.

Female social reformers and activists, on the whole, had independent financial means which obviated the need to earn a salary.[25] For the middle-class spinster with no means of financial support things were somewhat different. Financial need was her overriding concern, and her options were severely limited. Realistically, there were only two occupations to choose from, if an air of respectability was to be maintained. But with growing numbers of women chasing positions as governess or lady's companion, both were oversubscribed and underpaid. Issues of respecta-bility aside, the poor education most girls received left them ill-equipped to enter the wider job market (Vicinus 1985).

While middle-class boys went to school to be prepared for positions in the world of commerce or public service, middle-class girls' education, in mid-century, focused entirely on the skills necessary for their predestined position in society, as wives, mothers and managers of the domestic economy (Perkin 1993). This education was delivered either in the home, by mothers or governesses, or at small private schools, whose purpose was 'to inculcate the domestic ideal [and] polish the young lady through training in the social graces' (McDermid 1995: 107).

However, the rising numbers of unmarried middle-class women who needed to work sparked a new interest in girls' education (Gleadle 2001). The nascent feminist movement was attuned to these societal changes and began to speak out for equal educational opportunities (McDermid 1995). In 1850, the opening of the North London Collegiate Girls' School marked the beginning of a more intellectual approach to girls' education. Founded by educational reformer, Mary Frances Buss, it provided a rigorous academic education to the daughters of professional middle-class families. Cheltenham Ladies' College, which opened a year later, provided a similar style of education, but to a more socially elite group of girls. While a number of similar schools opened around the country, it should not be concluded that the Victorian middle class suddenly embraced education for their young women. By 1900, it is estimated that only 30 per cent of middle-class girls attended the new schools and colleges; the majority continued to be educated at home, or at old-style schools, whose focus on the acquisition of social skills rather than academic attainment persisted (Steinbach 2004).

Colleges providing training for specific occupations also began to emerge (Perkin 1993). In 1848, Queen's College (an Anglican institution associated with King's College, London) opened to train women as teachers and governesses. This was followed, in 1850, by Bedford College (later to become part of the University of London), offering a more liberal education, but still directed mainly at women wishing to become teachers (Steinbach 2004). The establishment of these colleges was of great importance in the development of academic education for women, but of even more significance was the campaign by a group of feminist reformers – including Barbara Bodichon, Emily Davies and Elizabeth Garrett Anderson – to open up women's access to higher education. As a result Girton College, the first women's college at Cambridge, opened in 1869, followed by Newnham in 1871; while at Oxford, Lady Margaret Hall and Somerville opened in 1879 (Steinbach 2004).

The search for respectable employment options for 'surplus women' was taking place at the same time that nurse leaders were developing nursing reforms, calling for better educated recruits and an improved social standing for the occupation. Putting these two problems together, one logical conclusion was that nursing should be developed into an occupation which appealed to single middle-class women. Central to nurse reformers' plans was the development of nurse training schools, and this objective chimed with the increasing interest in women's education. Middle-class women could be enticed into the hospitals by the offer of education and training, and their presence would boost respectability of the profession.

Nursing was thus refashioned as a respectable occupation, making extensive use of middle-class ideology, stressing the feminine nature of the work and its philanthropic and charitable overtones, and describing it in terms all too familiar to their target candidates. Provision of training addressed the new desire for education, and invocation of the family metaphor rendered hospitals as safe and quasi-familiar environments. The construction of a familiar set of relationships and hierarchies, and instillation of strict codes of discipline protected respectability, reassuring both recruits and their parents.

One barrier to respectability remained: the prohibition against paid work. The subject of pay for the 'new nurses' was considered controversial (Gamarnikow 1978; Vicinus 1985; Poovey 1989). For an occupation laced with connotations of devotion and self-sacrifice, the prospect of sullying this image with worldly reward was unappealing. Throughout the century some middle-class women continued to enter nursing on a voluntary basis, but such devotion was of little help to women who needed to earn a living. Reformers lobbied hard for pay for the new nurses, and the battle was won quite quickly

(Gamarnikow 1978). The steady increase in numbers of middle-class women moving into paid work of all sorts made it generally more acceptable to work for a wage, and this relaxing of social mores eased any residual controversy surrounding the payment of 'lady' nurses (Vicinus 1985).

At some hospitals, such as the HSC, the practice of using volunteer nurses to work as sisters, supported by paid ward nurses (as pioneered by the nursing sisterhoods), persisted into the 1880s. Catherine Wood, Lady Superintendent from 1878 to 1888, worked on a voluntary basis for most of her tenure (GOS/5/2/30, 5 April 1871; GOS/1/2/12, 28 June 1871). However, by the end of the decade, most other London hospitals *required* trained nurses to take a salary. From hospital managers' point of view, despite the financial cost, it was preferably for these women to be paid. As employees, rather than volunteers, the managers could exert much greater control over this new and challenging workforce.

Conclusion

The history of nursing, as written by early twentieth-century historians, claims that the aim of mid-nineteenth-century reforms was to create a respectable occupation for middle-class women; and that by the end of the nineteenth century working-class women had all but been excluded, at least from hospital nursing. Nightingale is frequently quoted as calling for a better class of nurse, but was she really striving for an occupation inhabited exclusively by middle-class women, or proposing that it should merely adopt character-istics associated with this class? Her admission that the ideal nurse probably did not exist, seems to support the latter. Pragmatically, considering the rapid growth in the hospital sector which occurred in the second half of the nineteenth century, there would never be a large enough supply of middle-class women prepared to enter nursing. Lower-class women remained essential to the service, and the task of new nursing was to train them in the habits and character of their middle-class sisters. As Rafferty has written: 'Reconstructing the order of health care presupposed reforming the charac-ters of the nurses themselves, for which training was the key' (1996: 21).

Equally, the desire for better educated nurses, expressed by many doctors and driven by the increasing complexity of medicine, could have been mistaken by modern historians for class-based selection. It has been assumed in many analyses that, in calling for better educated women to join the profession, reformers were using the term synonymously with middle-class. This may be a misinterpretation. Nightingale is recorded as saying that class was irrelevant and what mattered was education and character (Abel-Smith 1960; Rafferty 1996; Bradshaw 2000). By the last decade of the nineteenth century, by which time compulsory education and elementary schools had been in place for some time, it is possible that respectable working-class women, with a suitable level of education, would prove just as attractive to nurse recruiters as Nightingale's supposed ideal.

This is not to say that middle-class women did not enter nursing in increasing numbers. There is a mass of evidence to show that they did, but this was not necessarily at the expense of women with lower social standing. An alternative reading of the pursuit of respectability for nursing may be linked to the improved education of girls and to the opening up of a variety of forms of employment for young women. Nursing reformers were competing with other employers for young women with better levels of education and new aspirations, of all classes. The 'respectability agenda', while appealing to middle-class women, could also have made nursing attractive to ambitious working-class women looking for opportunities for social advancement.

In this study, the development of nursing in one London teaching hospital is examined in depth, in an attempt to question whether the ideals and ideology of nurse leaders were representative of the reality of Victorian nursing reforms. The book does not set out to make definitive statements about the rise of modern hospital nursing, but rather uses evidence discovered by deep mining of the archive, and a prosopographical methodology, to question traditional understanding of nurses in this period. Using this approach, details of nurses' careers have been uncovered which previously have been unrecorded. Following Kathleen Williams' argument that to build a history of nursing, it is necessary to start with the detail of everyday life, the book is written from the nurse's perspective and organized along the lines of a career path (Williams 1980). Themes addressed include changing trends in recruitment, development of training, the experience of being a nurse at St George's and the development of careers, within and outside the hospital. Data from studies of other hospitals have been used, wherever possible, to draw comparisons, and discussion of other types of nursing, such as district nursing and private nursing, are included for comparative purposes.

The study follows Amanda Vickery's suggestion that detailed investigation of a specific group will yield new insights into the character of its members, and has developed evidence in support of Christopher Maggs' contention that the image of the 'new nurse' stemmed more from rhetoric than reality. The results suggest that nursing at St George's diverged from this ideal in many respects, and this may also be true of other hospitals.

The discussion of nursing at St George's is situated in the wider context of the changing role of women in Victorian society. Nursing history, so far, has made only a small contribution to the larger subjects of women's history and women's work, as Barbara Mortimer has suggested (Mortimer 2005). Perhaps it has been ignored by these disciplines because nursing itself is considered mundane, too closely associated with domestic work, a subject also ignored to a great extent by labour and gender historians (Davidoff and Hall 2002).

By putting ordinary nurses under the microscope this book reveals the complexities of Victorian working women, their ambitions and their quest for independence.

Pen Portrait 1 Harriet Coster – Maid to Matron

This is the story of a woman who started her working life as a housemaid, but rose to the position of Matron at the prestigious St George's Hospital.

Harriet Connor, born in 1833, was the daughter of a gardener at Middlesex District Pauper Lunatic Asylum. She left home in her teens to work as a maid in Birmingham, where she met her first husband, a fellow servant. Quickly widowed, with one small daughter to support, she found work as a nurse at Essex County Asylum. After barely a year in Essex, she found a new job (and promotion), as Superintendent of the lying-in wards at St Pancras Workhouse. This was the turning point in Harriet's life. At St Pancras she met her second husband, workhouse surgeon William Coster. Their marriage (in 1859) scandalized the workhouse guardians, but Coster was a popular officer and the Vestry supported the couple. Harriet was even promoted to Matron of the female wards, and later credited with remodelling the infirmary's nursing arrangements. In 1862, the couple moved back to Hanwell (the scene of Harriet's childhood) when Coster was appointed Medical Officer to the Central London District School. A family followed, but Harriet's life was about to be shattered. In quick succession she lost two of her young children, and then her husband. By 1870, she was once again left to support herself and her five surviving children.

Harriet turned to what she knew best, and was appointed Superintendent of Nursing at St George's in 1872. She marked a distinct change in policy at the hospital, which had been toying with 'lady' superintendents. Harriet represented a return to the more traditional style of matron, albeit one with direct practical experience of nursing. She worked quietly, in the background, seldom appearing in the hospital records. But under her 25-year tenure, St George's became one of the first to establish a three-year nurse training programme. On retirement, *The Hospital* described Harriet as '[belonging to] the older school of nurses' and spoke of the 'pathos attaching to much of her life' (*H/NM*, 7 August 1897: 168).

Harriet's views on 'modern' nursing are hard to uncover. Her appointment as Nurse Honorary Secretary to the RBNA (on her retirement), suggests sympathy with the anti-registrationists. By this time the RBNA (originally established to promote registration) had been infiltrated by Burdett's supporters. On her appointment, Harriet received scathing criticism from Ethel Fenwick, who described her a poodle of the medical men on the Committee.

Harriet continued to take an active part in the business of the RBNA until her death in 1915, at the age of 82. By then all but two of her children were dead, and the survivors were both overseas. Her story is testament to the possibilities that a nursing career opened up to women from very humble backgrounds.

Sources: This brief biography is an extract of a longer version of Harriet's life, to be published in *Women's History Review* (Hawkins 2010).

2 'The majority are ladies, a great many domestics'[1]

The Victorian movement to transform nursing from a despised job for widows and old women into a respectable profession for young gentlewomen was supported by doctors, hospital managers, nurse leaders and even patients.[2] Its supporters used the image of the 'new nurse' relentlessly, contrasting it with the 'old nurse', in a classic example of Victorian dichotomy of ideas of womanhood. The 'new nurse' was young, respectable, well-educated and single; pure, morally unimpeachable and full of Christian virtue. The old nurse, by contrast, was old, slovenly and gin-sodden. The two images were so pervasive that twentieth-century historians have accepted them as true representations of reality. Brian Abel-Smith, regarded as the first to apply rigorous historical method to the history of nursing, nevertheless failed to challenge this image in any detail. More recently, historians have begun to question the image, looking for evidence which tests it in the records of individual hospitals. In this chapter, a close examination of the records St George's Hospital will explode this accepted picture of Victorian nurses, revealing it to be a myth of the highest order.

Christopher Maggs has argued that historians have focused too much on contemporary accounts of nursing in magazines and nursing handbooks in forming conclusions of its 'gentrification', ignoring (or overlooking) the actuality at the local level. He claims that, far from representing reality, the 'ideal nurse' was merely a tool, used by nurse leaders to assimilate the characteristics of 'ladies' into a new image for the emerging profession. While a small number of middle-class women (and a handful of low-ranking members of the aristocracy) became nurses, they were numerically insignificant (Maggs 1980). Furthermore, the rigid discipline which defined the new nurse's life, and the hierarchical nature of nursing, erased any differences in social standing, creating what he called an 'earnest class'; a grouping which 'transcended all other class definitions' (Maggs 1983: 22).[3] The records from provincial hospitals, on which Maggs based his comparative study, enabled him to investigate some elements of the 'ideal nurse', but did not provide any evidence on which to base an analysis of class. Consequently, in drawing his conclusions on the social structure of nursing, he was forced to rely on evidence from contemporary published sources, contrary to his own critique of previous historical analysis.[4]

Ann Simnet undertook one of the first studies of the social structure of nursing based on institutional records. In the nursing records of St Bartholomew's Hospital (Bart's) she found information concerning the occupations of nurse recruits' fathers. Such data could shed light on the social standing of such women before they entered the hospital, and indicated that at Bart's they did become progressively more middle-class in the period between 1881 and 1892 (see Figure 2.1).[5]

Increasingly, probationers came from families of professional men – dentists, clergymen and the military; indeed, by 1892 the daughters of working-class fathers (Classes III to V) were completely absent. Simnet's results seem to support the contention that, at Bart's at least, nursing had become the domain of the privileged classes, in direct contradiction to Maggs' conclusions.

However, Simnet concluded that London hospitals were the exception rather than the rule, and pointed out that her study focused on nurse recruits only. As many probationers did not join the hospital staff on completion of training, their impact on the social structure of the hospital's nursing department would have been slight (Simnet 1986). This implies that the main body of nursing staff at Bart's was working-class, but Simnet had no data to support this; and while providing some useful data, the study left many unanswered questions.

Unlike Maggs, who described nursing as a social melting pot, Jane Brooks has argued that, from the 1860s onwards, although both upper- and

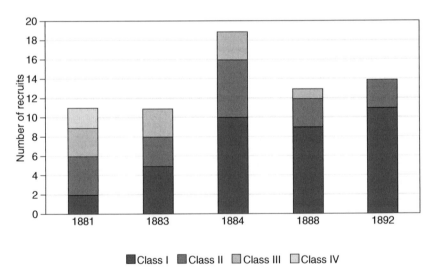

Figure 2.1 Analysis of class of nurse recruits at St Bartholomew's Hospital, 1881–92 (source: Simnet 1986).

working-class women were represented in the nursing workforce, the hierarchical structure permitted little movement between the two. Working-class women were recruited as ward nurses, while the upper and middle classes supplied the new hierarchy of sisters and matrons (Brooks 2001). This model is similar to the famous two-tier structure instituted at St Thomas' in the late 1860s, by Florence Nightingale and Mrs Wardroper.[6]

Support for the 'orthodox' view of the gentrification of nursing has been put forward by Janet Likeman, in her examination of nursing at University College Hospital (UCH). Like Simnet, Likeman used hospital records which contained details of fathers' occupations to assign social class to individual nurses, applying the Registrar General's scheme of occupational classification (Likeman 2002).

Her data indicate that the majority of nurse recruits at UCH came from the 'superior' social classes, and Likeman concluded that, by the end of the century, nursing had become an occupation dominated by single, middle-class women (2002; see Table 2.1). This is to ignore the large minority of recruits who came from Class III (the labour aristocracy). UCH was nursed by a sisterhood, and while not being unique in this, it cannot be said to be representative of nursing in London. As a result, Likeman's conclusion that nursing had become a vocation for upper- and middle-class women appears open to question.

The conflicting evidence as to class structure in nursing demonstrates the dangers of extrapolating the experience of one hospital to all hospitals. To test whether the occupation was heavily stratified according to class, as Brooks has suggested, or became a great melting pot, as Maggs has proposed, requires further analysis of nursing at yet more hospitals.

Much of the modern discussion on class in nineteenth-century nursing is complicated by a lack of clear definition of the terms which frame the debate. Historians must be aware of changing meanings over time of familiar words and their social connotations. Even Victorian commentators found themselves embroiled in semantic arguments regarding the definition of labels such as 'lady' or 'gentlewoman', terms used interchangeably by nurse reformers and their supporters. Consequently, historians are obliged to consider carefully what a writer was attempting to convey when such ambiguous terms were employed.

Table 2.1 Social class of nurse recruits at UCH, 1889–99

Class	No. of recruits
Class I	84
Class II	13
Class III	50
Class IV	15
Class V	3

Source: Likeman 2002: 39.

According to Rosalind Paget, founder of the Midwives' Institute and Trained Nurses Club, nursing was organized hierarchically, along class lines (Booth B154 (Paget), 8 May 1896: 18).[7] The posts of matron and sister were reserved for 'ladies', while lower positions (and private nursing) were the domain of the 'ladylike' (Booth B154 (Paget), 8 May 1896: 18). She defined what she meant by these terms:

> Trained nurses are drawn from the same class as nursery governesses, upper servants and shop girls and so-called gentlewomen, 'a non-descript class'. Gentlewomen are not Ladies they are the result of the levelling up and the levelling down process. ... Often daughters of the small professional classes.
>
> (Booth B154 (Paget), 8 May 1896: 18)[8]

Thus, Paget described nursing as a middle-class profession, with the upper classes holding positions of authority. Her view left no room for the working-class women encountered earlier in the century.

Paget's definition of what constituted a 'lady', as opposed to a 'gentlewoman', indicates that these terms were not clearly defined in Victorian society. A vigorous debate on the subject was conducted through a series of letters to *The Hospital* in the late 1890s, providing more evidence of their imprecise nature. A matron started the debate, complaining that, despite advertising for 'gentlewomen' to fill probationer posts in her hospital, she had been inundated by applications from 'all sorts and classes'. In her opinion, the term had implied 'good birth and education', but respondents had wilfully misunderstood this (*H/NM*, 6 August 1898: 167).

Some readers of *The Hospital* disagreed. According to one, who wrote as 'A Nurse', the term 'gentlewoman' referred to, 'women of refined and gentle manners, whose minds are pure and holy, no matter whether they be rich or poor, high born or low born, educated or uneducated' (*H/NM*, 13 August 1898: 174). Another wrote, somewhat confusingly, 'A true woman is a lady, and a true lady a gentlewoman; and every woman who behaves as such merits the treatment and respect of both' (Hill, *H/NM*, 20 August 1898: 183). A third stated that 'gentlewoman' described a state of mind and collection of behaviours, whereas 'lady' denoted birth and (sometimes) education: 'it is certainly possible for a woman to be a lady without being a gentlewoman' (Lear, *H/NM*, 27 August 1898: 191). All agreed that the term 'gentlewoman' referred more to a woman's manner of living than how or where she was born. As another wrote, 'The qualities which go toward the making of a gentlewoman ... can only be cultivated and developed ... real gentlewomen are recognised by their lives and not by their dress' (Brighouse *H/NM*, 27 August 1898: 191). In the view of these writers, it was the matron's understanding of the word which was misconceived, rather than that of her applicants.

However, she was not without support. According to 'XYZ', 'Gentle-woman means simply a woman of gentle birth.... Women of humbler origins can never lay claim to the title.' This writer also criticized the con-temporary usage of the term 'lady' which once had been synonymous with 'gentlewoman' but now, 'simply means a person of the feminine gender, being applied alike to the highest lady in the land and to the "laidy" who sweeps a crossing' (XYZ, *H/NM*, 20 August 1898: 183).[9]

This confusion over definitions highlights the problem of taking con-temporary reports of the gentrification of nursing at face value. When nurse reformers talked about introducing 'ladies' to the profession, were they referring to women of good birth, or rather, implying women of good education and exemplary character? Were they referring to real women at all? Or were such terms being used to create an association in the public's mind between nursing and the *qualities* they wished to be associated with the 'new nurse'?

This contemporary confusion over what constituted a 'lady' and a 'gentlewoman' was reflected in interviews with matrons conducted for the Charles Booth Survey of London. According to Isla Stewart, Matron at Bart's, her nurses were drawn from all sections of society, although the majority were 'middle class'. To illustrate this, she stated that at the time of the interview they had two daughters of baronets and two labourers' daughters among their ranks (Booth, B153 (Stewart), 8 April 1896: 60).[10]

Miss Monk, Sister Matron at King's College Hospital, claimed a wide range of social backgrounds for her nurses, but admitted that the majority came from the 'middle and domestic classes', that is, 'people who would otherwise be governesses or domestic servants'. Unlike at Bart's (which appeared to offer equal opportunities for promotion), at King's, the 'Sisters and Matrons are generally ladies, [coming from] county families.' Miss Monk continued, 'No woman can be a Sister here who is not gentle-woman born.' Despite this discrimination, all King's sisters were obliged to go through the same training regime as ordinary nurses (Booth, B153 (Monk), 9 April 1896: 82).

Miss Vincent, Matron at the St Marylebone Infirmary, also preferred 'middle class' women, who she described as the daughters of 'shop keepers, professional men [and] farmers'. Women from 'the servant class' were not admitted unless they proved to be 'particularly desirable'. (Booth, B153 (Vincent), 15 April 1896: 120).

The Assistant Matron at the Westminster Hospital (Miss Carwen) was not so dogmatic. Her nurses came from all classes she said, 'The majority ... are ladies ... daughters of clergy, lawyers and doctors ... and a great many [are] domestic [servants].' This confused reply could indicate Miss Carwen's dilemma in wanting to emphasize the refinement of the hospital, in order to attract high-calibre nurses and continued donations and sub-scriptions, while at the same time feeling obliged to be honest about the actual composition of the nursing staff, in an interview for such a prestigious study (Booth, B153 (Carwen), 18 April 1898: 158).

Agreeing with Miss Monk, the matrons from St Thomas' and the London Hospital (Miss Gordon and Miss Luckes, respectively) stated a preference for ladies as sisters (Booth, B153 (Gordon), 21 April 1896: 178; Booth, B153 (Luckes), 29 April 1896: 220). At St Thomas', only specials (lady probationers) were ever appointed as sisters, while Miss Luckes also preferred such women in that role. At St Thomas', the ordinary ranks of probationers were filled by the higher classes of servants and daughters of professional men; while many of the regular nurses at the London had been parlour maids, housemaids ('of the better sort'), or women who in 'former days' would have been governesses or music teachers. Only St Thomas' had completely separate schemes for paying probationers and ordinary probationers. Most other hospitals accepted paying probationers, but, to make a career out of nursing, they were obliged to join the ordinary trainees to complete training and obtain a full certificate.

The Booth interviewees often gave examples of the type of person they were referring to when mentioning class. The term 'middle class' was generally used to describe the daughters of doctors, clergy, military officers, shop keepers, professional men and farmers. 'Ladies' was sometimes used to differentiate a small group of women from the others, and could refer to 'county families' or women who were 'gentlewoman-born', as at King's. At other times though, it was used synonymously with the term 'middle class'. Miss Carwen used 'ladies' to mean the 'daughters of clergy, lawyers and doctors', whom Miss Vincent described as 'middle class women' (Booth, B153 (Carwen), 8 April 1896: 60).

The interviewees also described recruits in terms of what occupations they would have had in 'former days': governess, music teacher, 'failed' pupil teachers and parlour maids 'of the better sort' (Booth, interviews with matrons, B153, 1896).

By examining these responses, a clearer picture emerges of the social structure of nursing within London's hospitals at the end of the nineteenth century. The daughters of professional men (the 'middle classes') featured frequently in the interviews, and the interviewees gave particular weight to this group, always mentioning them first in their lists of preferred recruits. However, rather than reflecting a superiority in terms of numbers, the positioning of such women at the head of the lists may have served to create an impression that they dominated the nursing departments. Evidence for this desire to emphasize the middle-class nature of the profession might be drawn from Miss Carwen's conflicting statements, referred to above.

All but one of the matrons interviewed admitted that they accepted servants to train as nurses. It could be argued that hospitals were obliged to take such women in order to maintain staffing levels, in the face of a shortage of suitable middle-class candidates. This seems unlikely, however, given the repeated references in nursing journals to 'overcrowding' of the profession, and the overwhelming number of applicants for training courses. In the mid-1890s, Guy's reported over 2,000 applications annually, for only 70 places, while The London experienced similar interest in its training scheme (Morten 1892).[11] Given the volume of applicants, hospitals were able to select the very best candidates for the job, and despite the rhetoric, these may not necessarily have been women from privileged backgrounds. However, the middle-class recruits were emphasized by matrons to promote the respectability of the profession (and of the hospitals in which they worked). They may even have been window dressing, used to divert attention from the true picture – that women from the lower classes were being employed in large numbers.

Care needs to be taken in extrapolating the Booth interviews to the whole body of nursing in Britain at this time. Booth's interviewees represented London hospitals only, and, as Christopher Maggs has already observed, the situation in London was possibly quite different to that which pertained to the provinces.

In reality, it appears that the major hospitals in London recruited significant numbers of nurses from both the 'middle class' and the 'servant class', and that while 'ladies' were preferred as sisters at some, this was by no means universal. This picture seems to support Maggs' conclusions, from his study of provincial hospitals, that nursing had become a melting pot, taking all classes and ranks from society and blending them into a new hierarchy within the hospital (1980, 1983). Jane Brooks' argument that all classes in society were represented in the nursing profession but that the hierarchy of class was maintained within nursing departments, also finds some support (2001). However, Isla Stewart's comment that any nurse could become a matron, regardless of her background, indicates that this was not universal practice, and that some very influential nurse leaders contradicted it (Booth, B153 (Stewart), 8 April 1896: 60).

Preoccupation with the class of nurses was not restricted to London-based voluntary hospitals, but pervaded other emerging branches of nursing around the country. In district nursing, women of 'breeding' and education were deemed essential for work which involved not only patient care, but bringing order, cleanliness and morality into the homes of the poor. As Florence Lees (first Superintendent of the London Metropolitan and National Nursing Association) wrote, 'Nurses of the same class as the poor among whom they had to work, would not generally undertake the task of contending against dirt and disorder in [their] rooms' (quoted in Wildman 2009: 56). Her vision for district nursing mirrored reforms in hospitals, placing emphasis on education and training, 'making [district nursing] a profession fit for women of cultivation' (quoted in Sweet and Dougal 2008: 10).

There was a dimension to the class debate peculiar to district nursing. In the latter half of the nineteenth century, district (or home) nursing was offered by a wide range of providers: from the virtually untrained self-employed village 'handiwomen', through to trained nurses provided by private nursing institutions. Organizations, such as William Rathbone's Nurse Training Association in Liverpool and Lees' London-based association originally provided care for the deserving poor, but soon found that they could generate income by sending nurses into the homes of the upper classes (Sweet and Dougal 2008: 20). This triggered controversy as to what type (or class) of woman would be best suited to these very different roles: particularly, the expectation that rich private patients would demand nurses 'of refinement and scientific training' (Sweet and Dougal 2008: 23).

This assumption was not uniformly accepted. Philippa Hicks, superintendent of the Nurses' Cooperation, reported a great demand for the 'upper housemaid class' as private nurses amongst the social elite. (Booth, B153 (Hicks), 13 April 1896: 138).[12] She found the daughters of farmers or tradesmen the easiest to place. Ladies on the other hand were troublesome 'because it is hard to know what to do with them'. She found that the presence of lady nurses in upper-class homes confused the relationship between employer and employee, but they were also ill equipped to deal with the working classes in their own homes.

Within district nursing there was similar disagreement. Lees was in favour of encouraging 'the emerging professional class of women' into district nursing, in order to raise its status; whereas Rathbone preferred women recruited from similar backgrounds to the patients they would serve. According to Sweet and Dougal, 'this class tension underpinned the argument between the Queen Victoria Jubilee Institute for Nurses (QNI) in London and Rathbone's association in Liverpool', and continued well into the twentieth-century (2008: 10).[13]

A word of caution: as in the discussion of class in voluntary hospitals, most evidence for the class structure within district and private nursing has been drawn from the writings of nurse leaders or activists. Each had their own agenda to promote. It would be interesting to examine the membership of the QNI to see if it was as elitist as it portrayed itself.

These various accounts underline the difficulties in extrapolating results of local studies to form conclusions about nursing nationwide. Maggs has stressed the importance of local studies of nurse training, to counterbalance an historiography based on evidence from the writings of society's elite; but for such studies to be of use in understanding wider trends, further investigations are required to enable comparisons and conclusions to be drawn.[14]

None of the studies to date on the supposed gentrification of nursing have looked further back than the 1870s, to an era which marked the beginning of the reforms. By omitting the early years, these studies began when the trends they were attempting to track had already started to take effect. The base line from which they were emerging was thus undefined.[15]

One reason for this omission is a lack of records for these earlier years, and by relying on institutional archives alone, the studies have been restricted by this paucity of sources. Further, by using only probationer records, these studies have ignored other nurses, who may entered the hospital through other routes.

Lacking other evidence, conclusions about nursing in the mid-nineteenth century have continued to be based on the Sarah Gamp myth, and on contemporary reports of those closely associated with hospitals. Evidence such as that provided by John South, surgeon to St Thomas' Hospital, has been used by historians repeatedly to reinforce the Gamp image of pre-Nightingale nurses. He described nurses in 1857 'as much in the condition of housemaids and [requiring] little teaching beyond that of poultice-making ... and the enforcement of cleanliness and attention to the patients' wants' (Dingwall *et al.* 1988: 10).

Dr Steele, Medical Superintendent at Guy's, wrote of nurses at the hospital in the 1850s,

> For the ... appointment of nurse, which ... included not only attendance on the ... sick but the cleaning and scrubbing of the ward floors and of the staircases of the hospital, it was necessary to select from a class of inferior grade ... usually speaking, but little removed from the ordinary class of domestic servants.'
>
> (Steele 1871: 541)

Sisters, on the other hand, should be 'respectable females [with] ... experience of household work, [who had] been upper servants in private families'. It was not infrequent, he said, for sisters to be promoted from the ranks of ordinary nurses, based on length of service and suitability (Steele 1871: 541).

Clinton Dent, surgeon and nurse educator at St George's in the late nineteenth century, appeared to disagree with South and Steele. He defended the old nurses, asserting that, while lacking formal education, they were not ignorant women (Dent 1894b); and recent focus on early nurse reforms has also questioned the view of pre-reform nurses as ignorant old widows (Rafferty 1995; Summers 1989; Helmstadter 2002).

This chapter will address the changing social structure of nursing at St George's Hospital in London. Using the methodology described in Appendix 1, the backgrounds of nurses were investigated, and the changing structure of the Nursing Department between 1850 and the end of the century revealed.

St George's Hospital

St George's Hospital, one of the oldest voluntary hospitals in London, was founded in 1733. It arose out a schism within the Board of the

Westminster Hospital and the dissenting members (including all the medical staff) set up a new hospital in Lanesborough House, Hyde Park Corner, where it stayed for 247 years. The hospital was financed by subscriptions and donations (Blomfield 1933). Its purpose was to provide care for poor people who had suffered accidents or 'accidental diseases such as epidemic fevers' (SGHWB/53, 18 May 1870). Like all voluntary hospitals, its relief was targeted at the deserving poor, not at paupers (whose parlous condition was the result of their own actions). The hospital was managed by a Weekly Board of Governors, and any one of the hundreds of donors and subscribers was entitled to participate. The ultimate tier of management was the Quarterly Court, also open to all subscribers (Blomfield 1933).[16] It had aristocratic sponsors. The first president was the Bishop of Winchester, followed by the Prince of Wales, and during the period of this study, it was presided over by Queen Victoria herself. Subscriber lists contained the names of high-ranking nobles, politicians, clergy and military men.

With no elections to the Weekly Board, in practice, this left the hospital's management in the hands of a small coterie of interested parties (*The Times*, 7 January 1861: 8). The system came in for periodic attack. In 1860, a disgruntled governor described its financial management as being under the control of, '15 or 16 gentlemen who happen to be habitués of its weekly and quarterly boards ... the conduct of the hospital practically [resting] with a very small number of individuals, congregated by chance' (*The Times*, 16 July 1860: 12). In 1888, Timothy Holmes, (a surgeon at the hospital) defended its management, describing it as 'an open board in which medical men have by right a seat, but are in the minority' (Holmes 1888: 356). This arrangement was unusual. At other institutions, the management committee was composed entirely of laymen, and doctors had only an advisory role.

Occupying the same site for nearly 300 years, the hospital underwent many alterations and expansions. The most significant early development was the erection of a completely new building, in 1834, built behind, and replacing, the original Lanesborough House (see Plate 2).

Nursing at St George's, 1733–1850

When the hospital originally opened it had 30 beds and ten nurses. The Matron was regarded as the 'head of the family', housekeeper and enforcer of rules, and had little responsibility for the Nursing Department (Dent 1894a, 1894b, 1894c). In the earliest set of printed regulations, the Matron's responsibilities focus on control of the patients' behaviour and management of the hospital's supplies (SGHRO, 'Rules for Matron'). There were seven rules for 'Nurses', three of which concerned restrictions on movement. In one, the porter was instructed not to let any nurse out, 'under any pretence without leaving a ticket for that purpose signed by the Apothecary or Matron' (SGHRO, 'Rules for Nurses').[17] The rules give very little indication of the duties of the nurse, which appear to be restricted to policing the patients (especially with regard to the bringing in of 'victual or drink'), cleaning the wards and preventing outpatients from entering (SGHRO).

No reference was made to the type of women recruited, but the text of two advertisements provides some insight into eighteenth-century nurse profiles. In 1789, an advert in *The Daily Advertiser* called for, 'Any woman of fair character, in good health, between the age of 30 and 45 years, capable of discharging the office of Nurse ... particularly able to read writing [*sic*]' (Dent 1894b: 63). It seems that, even in the eighteenth century, the hospital managers wanted nurses with a certain level of education. A subsequent advert, in 1792, omitted the requirement for reading skills but gave more prominence to character, requiring the 'best testimonials for Sobriety and Diligence' signed by at least one housekeeper (Dent 1894b: 63). This seems to suggest that the ideal recruit would have been in domestic service. As nurses were expected to live in the hospital, they were probably either widows or single, although the presence of married women working as nurses cannot be completely ruled out. Taking this evidence together, the profile for an eighteenth-century St George's nurse was probably: aged between 30 and 45, without dependents, from a servant background, able to read, and physically capable of undertaking the duties of a nurse.

The hospital grew in size down the years, and the Nursing Department expanded, such that by 1834 there were 300 beds and 36 nurses (Dent 1894b).[18] In the early 1830s – possibly as a result of this growth in size (combined with disruption caused by building of the new hospital) – discipline was deemed to have become lax, and a new matron was recruited to introduce a stricter regime (Blomfield 1933). Authority over nurses' behaviour, and their hiring and firing (previously the preserve of the Weekly Board), was transferred to Mrs Steele. She was also tasked with keeping a record of women recommended as potential nurses, and vacancies within the Nursing Department were filled from this list (SGHWB/24, April 1836; SGHWB/25, 5 July 1837).

The new discipline proved too much for the nurses. In 1839, a committee investigating the high turnover of nursing staff found the 'new laws' had generated ill feeling among them. Relations with Steele had broken down, and the committee criticized her, stating she had 'not on all occasions shewn ... discretion with regard to temper' (SGHWB/25, 7 August 1839). They also accused her of failing to assess potential recruits' suitability on the grounds of health and 'medical qualifications' for the work (SGHWB/25, 7 August 1839).[19] A year later, after further disciplinary problems came to light, Steele resigned. In a long letter, she listed all the wrongs done to her, most particularly, that she had not had the support of the Board in instilling the strict rules they had hired her to impose.

After this incident, the governors reviewed the type of woman they considered suitable for the post of Matron. Their next advertisement requested applications from 'ladies with unexceptionable testimonials'. They should be unmarried, aged 30–45 and a member of the Church of England. There was no requirement for previous experience of hospital work. Of the 12 women who applied, eight may have been married or widowed. The application from Mrs Conway, who had a child aged ten, was accepted on condition that he be placed in a school should she be successful; but Mrs Forbes, whose living husband was in a lunatic asylum, and Mrs Wild, who also had a living husband, were both rejected (SGHWB/25, 17 February 1841).

Conway later withdrew from the process 'having ascertained that Mrs Haines had already secured the Votes and Interest of a very large number of Governors' (SGHWB/25, 24 February 1841). Canvassing governors was an accepted and expected tactic in securing a post; and Haines, who had prior knowledge of Steele's departure, took full advantage to all but secure the post before any other candidates had come forward (SGHWB/25, 24 February 1841).

She was duly appointed, and continued as Matron for eight years. She oversaw two developments of significance to the Nursing Department. In 1844, probationers from Elizabeth Fry's Society of Nursing Sisters were accepted to train as nurses. They spent two months on the wards, 'pledged to obey the Rules of the Hospital ... pay respect to the Matron and strict attention to Medical orders' (SGHWB/26, 27 March 1844).[20] There was no mention of fees being paid (either by the probationers or by the Society), but this event marked the beginning of a trail of women (as members of other nursing institutions or as individuals) entering the hospital to learn nursing. It also marked the awakening of the Board to the potential within its Nursing Department, to be a centre for training nurses for outside institutions.[21]

The second major development centred on night nursing at the hospital. Prior to 1849, head nurses had been the most senior members of the Nursing Department, followed by assistant nurses with night nurses occupying the lowest position. In common with other London hospitals, duties of the night nurse at St George's included cleaning the public areas of the hospital (such as the staircases and corridors) and the type of woman reflected that. They were employed on a casual basis, from groups who presented themselves each evening to be taken on for the night, often coming straight from other scrubbing or cleaning jobs (Helmstadter 1994).

In 1849, the Board at St George's was concerned about the quality of nursing at night. It decided to relieve night nurses of cleaning duties, and to elevate the role on to a par with head nurses. The change in status resulted in four of the existing staff being sacked and rehired as scrubbers. The rest assumed their new roles and were made responsible for their wards at night (SGHWB/27, 26 September 1849). In a further move to improve patient care at night, the hospital hired a nurse 'at a salary which will ensure the services of a superior person to act as Superintendent of the night nurses' (SGHWB/28, 13 April 1853). Head Nurse Harriet Richardson was appointed to the post, heralding the hospital's intention to promote existing staff to senior vacancies, rather than recruit externally (SGHWB/28, 13 April 1853; SGHWB/28, 22 June 1853). These changes to night nursing were innovative; St George's was the first to introduce the post of Night Superintendent, and possibly the first to introduce experienced nurses as night nurses (Helmstadter 1994).

Having been one of the first to employ experienced nurses to care for patients at night, St George's was one of the last to abandon the practice of maintaining a separate night staff (Helmstadter 1994). This system remained in place for 40 years, when difficulties in recruiting well-trained night nurses finally led the Board to decide that night nursing should be undertaken by all nurses, working on shift system (SGHWB/50, 6 April 1887).[22]

Growth of the Nursing Department

By the early 1850s, the Nursing Department had grown to 44, comprising 16 head nurses, 17 assistant nurses and 11 night nurses, and by 1884 it had

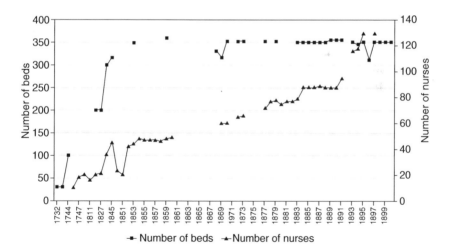

Figure 2.2 Number of beds compared to number of nurses at St George's, 1732–1900 (source: Data for 1732–1849: Dent 1894a, 1894b, 1894c. Data for 1850–60: St George's Hospital Nurses' Wage Books. Data for 1870–1900: St George's Hospital Weekly Board Minute Books and Committee of Nursing Minute Books. The sudden fall in numbers of nurses recorded in 1850 represents a transition from one source of data on nurse numbers to another, and is likely to be an anomaly between data sources, rather than representing an actual fall in nurse numbers).

doubled in size and continued to grow through the rest of the century (see Figure 2.2).

Prior to 1850, the number of nurses grew in line with the increase in beds; but from 1850, while bed numbers remained stable – despite the addition of three new wards – nurse numbers continued to rise. In an indication that St George's managers were beginning to heed developments in hospital design, the new wards added only one extra bed, and over the next 50 years the number of beds per ward fell from 13.3 to 11.9.[23] New understanding, particularly after the publication of John Erichsen's seminal work on the nature of hospital infections, defined a minimum cubic footage of space per bed, to ensure adequate ventilation and to prevent outbreaks of the dreaded 'hospital diseases' (Erichsen 1874).[24] Hospital managers responded to this growing understanding of the link between space and infection rates by adding extra wards but keeping the hospital's overall capacity static.[25]

As the number of beds stabilized, annual admissions underwent a slow but steady rise; the increased throughput of patients reflected in a fall in the average length of stay from 30.2 days in 1861 to 25.5 days in 1891 (Pinker 1966). One theory finds developments in medicine and improved nursing care at the centre of this phenomenon. But it has also been postulated that shorter stays resulted from an increasing demand for beds, stimulated by a surge of public confidence in the new scientific medicine (Woodward 1974). Hospitals struggled to meet the upsurge in demand, and this was certainly true at St George's. Earlier in the century, it had been claimed that over 1,000 patients, annually, were turned away or discharged early, through want of space (Dent 1894b).

Despite the relative stability in number of beds and patients, and the doubling in numbers of nurses during the period, the nursing reports for the whole period repeatedly state that it was 'undernursed'. This is illustrated best by the repeated references to rising costs of temporary nursing labour. When the Committee of Nursing produced its first Annual Report in 1877, it stated that 177 'special nurses' had been employed in addition to the regular staff of 73.[26] The 'specials' were requisitioned by the house physicians and surgeons to deal with difficult cases, which required one-to-one nursing (for fever and post-operative patients) or cases where 'male attendance was obviously desirable'.[27]

St George's expenditure on 'specials' (male and female) grew rapidly, the bill in 1877 being six times higher than it had been in 1870. Concerns were also raised regarding the reliability of outside nurses. The Resident Medical Officer (commenting on the use of 'specials') wrote in the 1884 Report that, 'The nurses trained here do the work in a much more satisfactory manner than those who have been trained elsewhere' (SGHWB/48, 26 March 1884). The fact that they also cost less probably did not go unnoticed.

To reduce reliance on outside staff, regular increases in the size of the

Nursing Department were authorized, by raising the number of probationers. This not only provided more nurses, but at the same time,
reduced overall expense, as probationers cost half as much as 'specials'
(SGHWB/47, 4 April 1883). In 1870, the first full year in which probationers were admitted, five entered the hospital and by the end of the decade
there were 13 on staff (SGHWB/24–61; SGHCON/1–2). Thereafter, the
number of probationers grew steadily, outnumbering head nurses by 1880,
and ward nurses by 1888. From this point on, it would be reasonable to say
that most of the bedside nursing was undertaken by probationers (see
Figure 2.3).

Despite nearly doubling the size of the nursing staff (it had reached a
total of 88 in 1888), it was still impossible to keep pace with the growing
number of 'special' cases, and in that year 319 outside nurses were used
(SGHWB/52, 10 April 1889). The problem persisted into the 1890s, when
the Weekly Board again voiced concerns, particularly regarding the
number of male nurses still being employed.

It is not clear why the number of 'special' cases increased so dramati-
cally during the 1880s. The introduction of anaesthetics (among other
medical innovations) enabled more complex cases to be admitted,
demanding more intensive nursing. Dr Steele commented that the
transfer to nurses of tasks such as care of tracheotomy and ovariotomy
cases (previously in the domain of medical students), had led to an
increased use of 'specials' in hospitals (*H/NM*, 26 February 1887). At St
George's, several new operating theatres opened in the early 1890s,

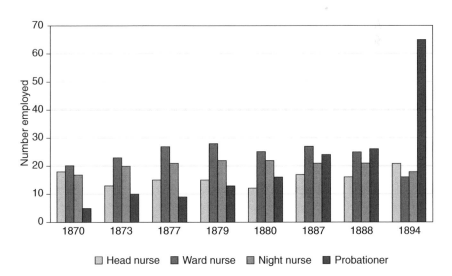

Figure 2.3 Growth in St George's Nursing Department, 1870–94 (source: St
George's Hospital Weekly Board Minute Books 1853–1900; St George's
Hospital Annual Reports. Dent 1894a, 1894b, 1894c).

suggesting an increasing number of operations were taking place with a resulting increase in demand for one-to-one nursing by 'specials' (SGHWB/53, 18 June 1890). External events, outside the control of the hospital, could also result in the use of higher than usual numbers of 'specials'. During the influenza epidemics in the early 1890s, for example, large numbers of nurses were rendered incapable of working, and specials had to be drafted in to fill their places (SGHWB/53, 1 April 1891).

By 1893, probationers accounted for over 50 per cent of the Nursing Department, and the strategy finally began to reap benefits. That year the number of extra nurses fell to 141 and after this date no further mention was made of them in the annual reports. Remarks about individual extra nurses continued to appear, however, indicating that their use did not die out completely.

The growth in size of St George's Nursing Department, during a period of stability in the number of beds and patients, can be explained (in part) in financial terms. By employing large numbers of probationers, reliance on expensive 'specials' could be reduced while maintaining an ability to respond in times of crisis. Probationers could cover experienced staff on routine cases, when the latter were required in cases of special need. This growing reliance on probationers, as the bedrock of the Nursing Department, also contributed to the lengthening of the probation period, from one year, initially, to three, by the end of the century. Increasing the number of probationers, and the duration of training, provided a readily available and cheaper solution to staffing crises.[28]

St George's was not alone in adopting this strategy. The Booth survey questioned metropolitan hospitals, with regard to the management and structure of their nursing departments. The results show that Bart's used

Table 2.2 Probationers as a percentage of nursing staff compared with patient:nurse ratios at various London hospitals, 1895–6

Hospital	Probationers as percentage of total nursing staff*	Patient:nurse ratio (1895)**
St Bartholomew's	76.1	2.2:1
The Royal Free	66.7	2.6:1
St Mary's	63.1	3.7:1
King's College Hospital	54.8	2.3:1
St George's	47.5	2.5:1
Guy's	46.2	2.3:1
Charing Cross	41.5	2.6:1
St Thomas'	31.7	2.5:1
The Middlesex	28.4	3.0:1
University College Hospital		2.1:1
The London		2.3:1
The Westminster		4.6:1

Sources: *Charles Booth Archive Hospital Questionnaires A27, pp. 24–134, 1896; **The Hospital 2 November 1895, p. 85.

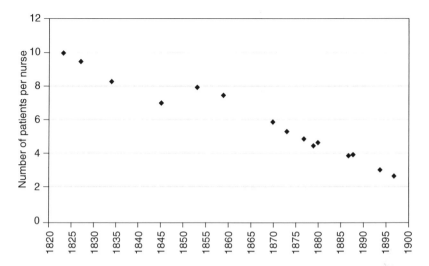

Figure 2.4 Patient:nurse ratio at St George's (source: St George's Hospital Minute Books and Committee of Nursing Annual Reports).

this strategy to the extreme, with probationers representing over 70 per cent of its nursing staff, while at Guy's and St George's the figure was just below 50 per cent (see Table 2.2).

In addition to the financial benefits, increasing the number of probationers enabled the hospital to reduce significantly the patient:nurse ratio (see Figure 2.4). During the 50 years of this study, this ratio declined rapidly at St George's from a high of ten patients to every nurse in the 1820s, to below three patients to each nurse by the end of the century.

According to *The Hospital*, in 1895, St George's patient:nurse ratio was on a par with the other major hospitals, being slightly better than Charing Cross and the Royal Free, but worse than Guy's, Bart's, King's College, the London and University College. As the data in Table 2.2 indicate most London hospitals were achieving good patient:nurse ratios by staffing their nursing departments with probationers. *The Hospital* suggested that a ratio of three patients to every nurse was 'not a high average ... but where the average falls below this, too large a preponderance of the unskilled element may be suspected' (*H/NM*, 2 November 1895: 85). The figures in Table 2.2 bear that out. The other danger inherent in this practice was the stress of 'exceptional severity' it placed on the senior nurses, supervising such large numbers of inexperienced workers (*H/NM*, 2 November 1895: 85). *The Hospital* concluded that low ratios of patients to nurses did not necessarily translate into either good patient care, or better conditions for the nurses themselves.

The article also showed that patient:nurse ratios were generally inferior outside London. It argued that, rather than reflecting low investment in nursing in the provinces, this disparity resulted from the intense competition which existed between London institutions, driving them to accommodate as many probationers as possible.

The reduction in the patient:nurse ratio at St George's reflected the frequency with which the Weekly Board was lobbied for increases in nursing staff by the Committee of Nursing (which in turn was lobbied by the Superintendent of Nursing and the medical officers). One of Florence Smedley's first actions as Matron was to demand an additional 25 nurses 'to improve the efficiency of the hospital' (SGHWB/60, 9 November 1898). Her request was rejected, but a few months later she again petitioned for 'staff nurses from outside the hospital' (SGHCON/2, 3 July 1899). In Smedley's eyes, the Nursing Department was still inadequate to meet the demands of an increasingly technical medicine and the clamour for treatment from the public.

Recruitment

By 1891 there were nearly 10,000 hospital beds in London and a falling patient:nurse ratio in all hospitals (Pinker 1966). The demand for nurses was enormous, but there was no shortage of potential recruits. Nursing departments at all major London hospitals were oversubscribed, and by 1897 St George's was refusing 600 applicants annually, while other hospitals received hundreds of applicants for each vacancy (see Table 2.3).

Table 2.3 Applications for places on probationer training schemes at London hospitals in the mid-1890s

Hospital	Applications
St Bartholomew's*	Nursing is increasing enormously and the number of candidates is much greater than it was.
Nurses Cooperative*	Nursing is considerably overstocked
Westminster Hospital*	1,000 applicants for 25 vacancies annually
St Thomas'*	2,500 applicants for 45 places annually
The London*	2,000 applicants for 150 places
St George's⁺	600 refused annually
Guy's⁺	2,500 applicants for 70 places
The Middlesex⁺	Several refused daily
Manchester Royal Infirmary⁺	400 applicants for 30 places
Liverpool Royal Infirmary⁺	Large number refused annually

Sources: *Charles Booth Archive Booth B153; ⁺ Morten 1892.

The project to turn nursing into a respectable profession for young women had reaped its rewards, to such an extent that it had acquired 'fashionable' status. A nurse writing in *The Daily News* said 'I am not one of those persons who go into hospitals for the sake of ... being fashionable' (*Daily News*, 3 January 1889: 3). Another wrote that 'the tide of applicants queuing up for training is a result of a change in fashion', while *The Hospital* criticized the 'kinds of girl [who] join nursing wilfully, out of fashion' (*Standard*, 9 March 1889: 2; *H/NM*, 20 August 1892). The fashionable status of nursing was wielded by many critics against the modernizers and their objectives.

By the end of the century, the existence of manuals, providing advice to prospective probationers indicates the level of interest in the occupation. Honnor Morten's, *How to Become a Nurse and How to Succeed* ran to at least three editions in the early 1890s, while Henry Burdett (doyen of hospital administration) edited a similar book, which was published into the twentieth century.[29] Both offered a career guide to aspiring nurses, including sections on how to apply, details of hospitals' conditions of employment, characteristics of a successful nurse, what to expect from probation and opportunities for qualified nurses.[30]

The high demand for nurse recruits was not restricted to the later years of the nineteenth century. At times, St George's needed to recruit the equivalent of nearly 50 per cent of its entire Nursing Department every year (see Table 2.4). This early recruitment was not driven by organic growth in the Nursing Department, however, but had its roots in an exceptionally high turnover in nursing staff pre-1870.[31]

The remainder of this chapter will consider what evidence, if any, can be found in the burgeoning Nursing Department at St George's to support the supposed gentrification of nursing, discussed earlier. Was there a dramatic shift in the social constitution of the Department between the 1850s and the end of the century, or did it remain essentially the preserve of working-class women?

Unlike previous studies on social class and nursing, which relied on information from hospital archives, this study used decennial censuses to locate details of nurses' families. The result was a much broader coverage

Table 2.4 Recruitment of nurses at St George's Hospital, 1850–99

	Average no. of recruits per year	Average staff size	No. of annual recruits as per cent of staff size
1850–9	23	49	48
1860–9	16	60	27
1870–9	35	73	48
1880–9	28	84	33
1890–9	33	116	29

Source: St George's Hospital Archive: Weekly Board Minutes; Registers of Nurses.

of the whole nursing staff, not restricted to probationers, as in other studies. Census information was combined with archival data to create brief biographical profiles of St George's nurses, and the resulting profiles enabled the change in a range of characteristics within this group of women to be investigated, over the period 1850 to 1900.[32] The characteristics studied include social class, age on joining, impact of family background on career prospects, geographic origin of recruits, previous work experience, marital status and family connections.

Analysis of social class[33]

A clear pattern in the changing social profile of the St George's nurses emerged, as the percentage of nurses from Classes I and II underwent significant growth throughout the period, particularly in the final decade (see Figure 2.5). In interpreting these data, it should be noted that information for 1852–71 was sparse, compared to other decades. This is partly the result of the missing census return for 1861 (destroyed by fire many years ago), but also reflects the relative size of the Nursing Department in those years, compared to the end of the century.[34] The

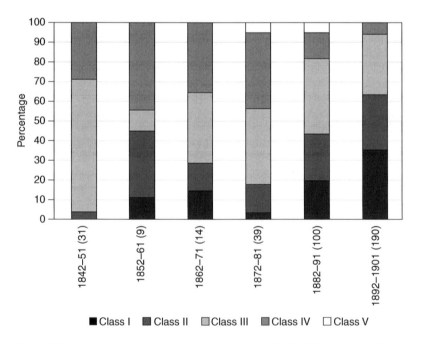

Figure 2.5 Social class of nurses at St George's, 1840s–90s (source: St George's Nurses' Database. The data have been organized according to date of start of the nurses. For some nurses this was not known, and their date of start was assumed to be in the ten years prior to the census in which they appeared).

comparatively large proportion of nurses coming from Classes I and II during 1852–71 should therefore be viewed with caution – the total population sample for these decades being only nine and fourteen, respectively – and of those, five were matrons. If the data for these two decades is ignored, then a clear progression can be seen from the 1840s to the end of the century, as Classes I and II increase steadily in proportion to the rest.[35]

As in Simnet's study from Bart's, Classes I and II represent the upper and middle classes, Class III, the skilled working classes (or labour aristocracy) and Classes IV and V the semiskilled and unskilled working classes, respectively.

Fathers' occupations of nurses in Class I were dominated by the church, the military, medicine and the legal profession. There were also a number of industrialists. In Class II the predominant occupations were farming and teaching, followed by small business owners and dealers in commodities. In Class III the fathers were tradesmen – carpenters, bakers, grocers and plumbers; but the largest group of women in this class were classified according to their own previous experience as nurses or cooks.[36] In Class IV, most women were also classified according to their own prior employment, usually domestic service. The fathers of nurses in Class IV tended to be agricultural labourers, while the few from Class V were general labourers. Assigning nurses to Classes III, IV and V was more likely to have been based on their own previous experience, as women from these classes were more likely to have worked prior to entering nursing.[37]

By the end of the century the proportion of nurses from Classes I and II rose from under 5 per cent (in the period 1842–51) to just under 60 per cent. Nurses from Class III represented at least one third of the total throughout, while nurses recruited from Classes IV and V dropped to under 10 per cent, having accounted for 40 per cent of the workforce in the period 1872–81. The relatively high proportion of nurses in Class III compared to IV, in 1842–51, could be explained by such women being classified according their own previous employment, rather than that of their fathers. Many of the nurses in this decade had previously worked as nurses or cooks, which placed them in Class III. Some of these women could have come from more humble backgrounds and the relatively large numbers in Class III would then reflect a degree of upward mobility.

The extent of social mobility in Victorian England is poorly understood. According to Jose Harris, the most 'open and frequently traversed' class barrier was between the upper working and lower middle classes, in which she includes teachers and clerical workers (Harris 1994: 8–9). F.M.L. Thompson disagrees, and claims that 'occupational mobility' within the working classes, rather than between working and lower middle classes, was the more common (1988: 83). Although not agreeing about its nature, both historians concur that social mobility existed in some form in

Victorian society. It is possible that St George's nurses of the mid-nineteenth century saw nursing as an opportunity to improve their social standing. This may also be true later on. As the social status of nursing improved (as a result of the modernizers' activities) it is plausible that working-class women would see nursing as route to social advancement.

The growth in numbers of women from Classes I and II, and the gradual disappearance of those from Classes IV and V, confirms an increasing gentrification of the Nursing Department at St George's Hospital. However, by the 1890s, with just under 40 per cent of its staff still originating from Classes III and below, it cannot be said that the hospital had become an exclusive bastion of middle-class nursing.

The two-tier structure of nurse training (designed to recruit a 'better class' of nurse and pioneered at St Thomas') has already been discussed. Such schemes differentiated between 'paying' or 'lady' probationers, and ordinary probationers, who were generally paid during their training. By the end of the century, similar schemes had been introduced at most London hospitals, with the exception of the Westminster and St George's.[38] Why had St George's not followed this trend – which on the face of it conveyed many benefits?

No mention of paying probationers is made in the records until 1895, when the Committee of Nursing approved the admission of such women, subject to suitable rules being compiled (SGHCON/2, 14 January 1895). The rules did not materialize until 1897, when they were finally published in the Committee's minutes, but paying probationers still failed to appear in the Nurse Registers (SGHCON/2, 18 January 1897). There is also no record in the accounts of any money having been received. This absence is made even more significant by the inclusion, in the early 1890s, of a very small income generated by the hospital's weekly lectures on nursing. The fact that these monies were recorded adds weight to an interpretation of the absence of training fees as evidence for the absence of paying probationers.

Despite the apparent lack of a paying probationer scheme, St George's was able to attract women from the higher social classes, and it is highly probable that, unlike neighbouring institutions, such women were treated no differently from their socially inferior colleagues. They are included in the Nurse Registers alongside nurses from more lowly backgrounds, with no distinguishing comments. If the hospital did accept paying probationers in the late nineteenth century, no record has survived.

The issue is discussed in more detail in the following chapter, but it seems to be reasonable to assume that the hospital never established such a branch of its Nursing Department, in the nineteenth century at least.

This is not to say the subject of lady nurses was never discussed.[39] Over the years, St George's considered various proposals to introduce lady nurses (as opposed to paying probationers) into the hospital. In 1857, the Board was approached by Lord Percy who presented the case of 'an

English Lady' wishing to take over the whole nursing of the hospital 'at her own expense' (SGHWB/30, 21 October 1857). The Board, tempted by her offer (and its financial implications) suggested she be allocated a number of wards as an experiment. Simultaneously, a survey of London hospitals was ordered, to reveal any experience of similar schemes. The only hospital which had tried such a scheme was King's, 'where a few ladies were employed as superintendents or head nurses'. Their experience was reported as satisfactory, and St George's decided to proceed with its own experiment, subject to the lady in question being 'suitably qualified for the job' (SGHWB/30, 4 November 1857).[40] This was the last entry on the subject in the Minute Books and it is assumed that the experiment never took place: whether because the lady proved unsuitable or because she withdrew her offer is not known.

The idea of ladies managing the wards would have been attractive to the hospital's governors on several levels. They might have hoped such women would inculcate a new level of discipline among the nurses and patients.[41] The minutes of the Weekly Board meetings were littered with references to unacceptable behaviour among both groups, especially in the early years of this study. Patients were reported for smuggling food and drink into the wards (expressly forbidden by hospital rules) and attacking nurses and other patients, verbally and physically. In one particularly violent case, a mother visiting her sick child was reported to be in 'liquor & in an excited state, having put her fist into the face of a young woman in an adjoining bed' (SGHWB/33, 12 July 1865). It could be expected that the presence of lady nurses might temper this behaviour.

Squabbling amongst nurses and patients was common, as was arguing with doctors, board members or the Matron. The frequency with which arguing and complaining was reported gives an impression of a very vocal workforce, unafraid to speak its mind, quite unlike the 'ideal' nurse who was quiet, obedient and modest. The presence of lady nurses, with their middle-class propriety and superior moral influence, was expected to eradicate such unacceptable behaviour and smooth the rough character of the regular nurses and patients. They were also expected to bring another advantage to the hospital: their willingness to work on a voluntary basis, and even to bear the financial load for all the nursing.

It is no coincidence that St George's continued to pursue the idea of lady nurses into the 1860s. A major review of the hospital's financial position in 1860 revealed a worrying position. Although it had several large legacies, worth £2,000 annually, a property portfolio which generated in the order of £3,750 per annum, and subscriptions worth £4,000, its expenditure was running at £16,000 a year. An aggressive fund-raising campaign was immediately launched to increase donations and subscriptions (SGHWB/31, 14 March 1860).[42] At the same time, the Board cast around for options to reduce costs, and it is not surprising that nursing – as the largest department in the hospital – was identified as an area for potential savings.[43] Lady nurses, working on a voluntary basis, offered a very attractive solution.

In 1860 (three years after the original plan failed) the St John's House Sisterhood was asked to take over nursing at the hospital. Despite initial interest by the Sisters, this plan also collapsed when agreement could not be reached regarding the management of nursing services.[44] Undaunted by this second failure, the governors continued to toy with the idea of 'lady nurses'. In January 1866, a committee consisting of governors, the senior physician and the senior surgeon was set up to investigate the 'system of nursing now pursued in the Hospital'.[45] It recommended an experiment be tried, of placing the nursing in one or two wards under sisters from St Peter's House (SGHWB/33, 21 March 1866).[46]

The idea received almost unanimous support from the Weekly Board. The committee's reasons for selecting St Peter's House illustrate the delicacy of the proposal:

> [the Sisters have] no other commitment to public nursing which could conflict with their duty to St George's ... the peculiarity of dress and discipline are not so marked as in other cases ... [and] St Peter's House is under the immediate and direct supervision of the Bishop of London.
>
> (SGHWB/33, 21 March 1866)

As discussed in Chapter 1, sisterhoods were regarded with some suspicion, particularly when they became involved in public office, such as nursing. The stress placed by the committee on the involvement of the Bishop of London was important, as it aligned the sisterhood directly with the established Church, rather than an evangelizing sect, or even more troubling, an order which aspired to Roman Catholicism. Issues of divided loyalties (between the head of the sisterhood and the hospital authorities) would have concerned the committee; as would concerns that the general public would associate the distinctive dress worn by religious nursing sisters with religious zealotry. As St George's nurses did not wear a uniform at this time, the nursing sisters, in their semi-ecclesiastical dress, would blend uneasily into the fabric of the hospital.[47]

A further concern centred on the possible negative effect of the presence of a sisterhood on donors and subscribers. It would be very easy for potential supporters holding different religious beliefs (even within the Anglican communion) to be antagonized by such a move. In fact, in the same year as the St Peter's House plan was being discussed, the St John's House sisterhood took over the nursing of Charing Cross Hospital and subscriptions were cancelled in protest against suspected 'Romanism' (Summers 1989: 379). St George's governors must have followed developments at Charing Cross closely, taking warning from these events.[48]

The Bishop of London attempted to reassure St George's governors.

He commended the St Peter's House sisters strongly, 'both in reference to their zeal in the discharge of their duties and their obedience to himself', hoping to remove any apprehensions 'which may exist as to the adoption in a Hospital supported by voluntary contributions of such an experiment' (SGHWB/33, 21 March 1866). Seemingly satisfied with the bishop's support, the Board proposed that the nursing sisters should take over two contiguous surgical wards, which would keep the experiment contained within a specific, well-defined area. The sisters required only board and lodging, while the under nurses (who were not sisters) would be paid at the same rate as existing staff (SGHWB/33, 21 March 1866).

The proposal was presented to a Special Court of Governors, but faced a stream of objections and was rejected. While acknowledging the hard work done by the committee, the Court concluded, 'It does *not* appear desirable to ... [entrust] the nursing of the certain wards to the Sisters of St Peter's House' (SGHWB/33, 20 April 1866; original emphasis). Instead, a motion was laid before the Court that, 'the Committee be requested to consider and report upon the means of introducing into the hospital a training system for nurses, with the assistance of a Committee of Ladies' (SGHWB/33, 20 April 1866). This motion was passed by a large majority, and marked the end of another attempt to introduce lady nurses to the hospital.

The reference to a committee of ladies is one of the few pieces of evidence in the records which indicates the involvement of lady visitors in the hospital. Given its location, adjacent to Buckingham Palace, surrounded by royal parks and in the middle of the affluent area of Belgravia, it is hard to imagine that it did not attract a large number of ladies to help its cause (see Plate 3) A report on lady visitors, published in 1859, provides the only direct evidence that such women did participate in some way, but there is little information as to their role.[49] If a committee of ladies to oversee the introduction of nurse training was ever established, its activities were never reported to the Weekly Board.

The decision to recruit a Lady Superintendent – to replace the existing Matron – was the most important outcome of the Special Court of 1866. She would be 'a lady of education,' and most importantly, 'practically acquainted with hospital nursing' (SGHWB/34, 29 January 1868). The title of the role was changed almost immediately to Superintendent of Nurses.[50] This avoidance of labels associated with class could illuminate the hospital's attitude towards social hierarchies within its midst. Although women from higher social classes were admitted in increasing numbers, they were never differentiated from the others, either by title or by special privileges. This is in contrast to most other London hospitals, where terms such as lady pupil or special probationer, in addition to lady superintendent, were in common use. Such women often enjoyed separate accommodation (be it sitting rooms or sleeping quarters), worked shorter hours, or attended more advanced lectures.[51] The ethos of St George's appeared to be more egalitarian. Its reasons for taking this approach are hard to understand; given the location of the hospital, it might have been supposed that St George's would have been very conscious of the class of its nurses. However, several explanations for this unexpected attitude are possible, supported by evidence from the minute books, including an unfortunate early experience with a paying probationer.

In 1868, a 'lady' named Emily Jones, 'anxious to learn nursing', was introduced to the hospital, by surgeon Charles Hawkins (SGHWB/34, 2 September 1868).[52] Unlike most ladies who came for a few hours each day, for a short period of time, Jones wanted to live in the hospital and was prepared to pay for her board and lodging. In her apparent eagerness to please, she also offered to pay for the furniture in her room, which she graciously said could become the property of the hospital when she left. The Weekly Board may have felt insulted by this offer, as their reply was terse and ungracious: 'as far as furniture is concerned, all the rooms provided for nurses already have furniture in them' (SGHWB/34, 16 September 1868).

Jones could be regarded as St George's first (and probably only) paying probationer. But if the Governors harboured ideas about a new stream of income from such women, their experience with Jones may have served as a warning. Admitted in November 1868, she almost immediately suffered a severe breakdown and her friends were asked to 'take the most immediate measures consistent with all delicacy for her early removal from the hospital' (SGHCON/1, 18 November 1868).[53] The Board was obliged to repay her fees. The precarious nature of this form of income was revealed to the hospital's managers; and questions may also have been raised about the suitability of such women for nursing. Furthermore, her requests regarding her room may have been interpreted as an indication of the 'special treatment' such women might expect, especially if they paid a fee for their training.

In 1869, the Board finally recruited a Lady Superintendent. The experience may have achieved nothing more than to strengthen their suspicion of lady nurses generally. It was an odd appointment, given the recent rejection of sisterhoods, as Zepharina Veitch had trained under the All Saints Sisterhood at UCH, and prior to joining St George's had been a sister at King's.[54] Even before she had taken up the post, there were several confrontations with the Weekly Board. The first concerned her title: she wished to be known as Sister Ina. This request was flatly refused on the grounds that she might be taken for a religious sister. She defended herself in a letter to the Weekly Board which culminated in an offer to stand down:

> Since my appointment as Superintendent of Nurses ... 'a very uncomfortable feeling' has been excited by my asking to be called Sister ... [and] I should like fully to explain my request ... I think the Nurses would have a more friendly feeling to one whom they called 'Sister'

than one who they address by so common a title as Miss ... Mr Niven seemed to think I must be ritualistically inclined ... [and] his remarks have left a painful impression on my mind ... If the Committee feel so uncomfortable regarding my appointment, I am quite willing to free them from 3 months notice.

(SGHCON/1, 20 November 1868)

She stressed that she harboured no desire to form a sisterhood within the hospital; but, given that she had been trained by one, the Board's suspicions were understandable. Veitch was dismayed by the reaction to her request and pressed upon the Board her need for their support:

The entire *trust* [original emphasis] and help of the Nursing Committee [is essential], in what must be such arduous work for some time ... I dare not undertake the responsibility of the position unless I feel assured that [the Committee] thoroughly believe I am only what I profess to be, a thorough & staunch member of the Church of England, with no tendencies to ritualism in any form.

(SGHCON/1, 20 November 1868)[55]

Veitch often returned to her theme of the arduous nature of the office and the support she needed to carry it out successfully. She wrote again before she had even taken up the role, complaining of the rooms assigned to her:

I am fully alive to the fact that my position must, for some time at least, be one of great anxiety & fatigue, to which the necessity of inhabiting temporary & unsuitable rooms would ask more than I am sure the Committee would wish to put upon me.

(SGHCON/1, 11 January 1869)

And there were further requests: for water to be laid on to her rooms, for a water closet on the same floor and for a female servant to wait on her (SGHCON/1, 18 January 1869).

This stream of demands, questioning the Board's authority and judgement are in stark contrast to letters from previous matrons, such as Mrs Steele. None of these preparations had been necessary prior to the arrival of other matrons, and it is likely that the Board began to question, even then, if the benefits of a lady superintendent might be outweighed by the disadvantages. The experience may also have coloured their view of admitting ladies in any other roles, including as paying probationers.

Veitch stayed at the hospital only nine months, but in her short tenure she introduced uniforms for the nurses and admitted the first ordinary probationers (in April 1869). Her resignation, when it came, was accepted unanimously (and without debate) by the Board. They appeared relieved.

Veitch's appointment had been motivated, in part, by a desire to improve the social standing of the Nursing Department. In a letter to *The Times*, written shortly after her resignation, the writer praised St George's as one of only a small number of hospitals which had placed their nursing department in the hands of a group of ladies (*The Times*, 1 November 1869: 5). The hospital seemed to have found the whole experience uncomfortable. Nevertheless they persisted with the idea, replacing Veitch with Maria Gregory, daughter of a Surrey gentleman-farmer who had worked at the hospital for several months before the Superintendent's resignation. At the time of her appointment Gregory was 29 – under age for a job with a lower age limit of 30 – and consequently was not confirmed in position for seven months. During her short tenure as Superintendent of Nursing, there were several outbreaks of discontent among the head nurses, suggesting that the young Miss Gregory experienced some difficulty in commanding the respect of the older and much more experienced women who in theory worked under her.[56] She remained less than two years. No reason was given for her departure, but her request for testimonials suggests that she expected to continue to work in some capacity or other (SGHCON/1, 4 and 26 March 1872).

The experience with Veitch, and to a lesser extent Gregory, seemed to influence the Board's view on lady nurses, and the next head of the Nursing Department presented a very different profile from that of the two previous incumbents. Mrs Harriet Coster, who retained the post for 25 years, was a self-made woman. The daughter of a gardener at Hanwell Asylum and widow of Dr George Coster (late Medical Officer to the Hanwell Schools Board), she had gained her nursing experience working as Superintendent of Wards at St Pancras Infirmary.[57] Her recruitment signals that the hospital – abandoning its brief dalliance with lady nurses – had placed practical experience above social position, and age above idealistic youth. As a widow, with children to support, Coster was dependent on her income; to the hospital, therefore, she presented as a woman with practical experience gained in a tough environment, combined with a financial situation likely to render her more pliant than her two predecessors.

Having decided not to follow the emerging fashion for lady nurses the Board, while still determined to improve the quality of its Nursing Department, resolved that all nurses, regardless of class, should be treated the same.

Social class and hospital hierarchies

While Figure 2.5 illustrates the gradual increase in nurses from Classes I and II, it gives no indication of how social class might affect the ultimate position a nurse could achieve. The data for St George's have been analysed to investigate whether it followed the trend at other London

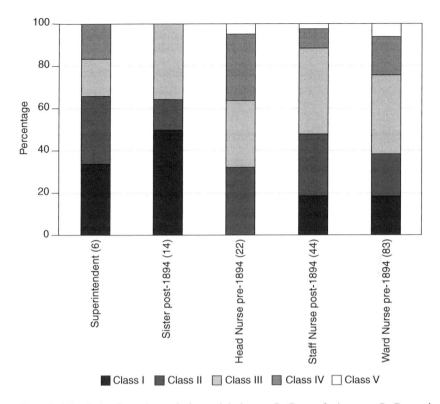

Figure 2.6 Analysis of nursing role by social class at St George's (source: St George's Nurses' Database).

hospitals, which restricted access to senior jobs to the higher social classes. Figure 2.6 charts the highest position achieved by a nurse during her career at the hospital, analysed by social class.

The family backgrounds of six of the eight matrons or superintendents of nursing (for the period of this study) have been traced. Perhaps not surprisingly, all but two were from Classes I and II. Harriet Coster's humble beginnings placed her in Class IV, and Hannah Kyle (Matron immediately before Miss Veitch) had first been found working as a dress-maker, which placed her in Class III. The position of the other senior role, that of sister (or head nurse), was not so straightforward.

A comparison of head nurses recruited before and after 1894 (when a major reorganization of the Nursing Department was implemented) shows a distinct gentrification taking place. Before 1894, 60 per cent of head nurses were working-class, while post-1894, the same percentage came from Classes I and II. Although St George's did not operate a 'lady proba-tioner' scheme, it seems that after 1894, women from the upper classes were preferred for promotion. What happened to produce this striking turn around? Closer inspection of the data reveals that sisters appointed between 1894 and 1897 (when Coster was still in charge) were evenly spread amongst the classes, and were all recruited internally. It is only after 1897, under Florence Smedley, that the balance shifted.[58] Seven of nine appointees came from the two upper classes, and all but one were recruited externally. Smedley's arrival was the catalyst for change, favouring privileged women for the first time. Her previous experience may have influenced her decisions at St George's.[59]

Lower down the hierarchy, social class appears to have been less important. A slight shift towards the upper classes is discernible in the comparative profiles of staff nurses and ward nurses (reflecting the changing intake of probationers), but women from Classes III to V predominated, in both periods.

The analysis of the changing social profile of nurse roles has been limited by small populations, but the large volume of data for probationers makes this group an exception. Figure 2.7 shows the changing social class of probationers joining the hospital, between their introduction in 1869 and the end of the century. Low numbers in the 1870s make conclusions for this decade contentious, but the much larger population of probationers in the 1880s and 1890s enable analysis.

From the moment the hospital admitted probationers, they were recruited from a broad range of social classes. In the 1870s and 1880s, Classes I and II represented 40 per cent of all recruits, but by the 1890s this proportion had risen to nearly 60 per cent. Nevertheless, even by the end of the century, in the decade which was supposedly dominated by the

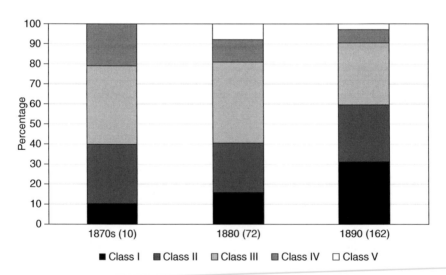

Figure 2.7 Analysis of social class of probationers at St George's, 1870–1900 (source: St George's Nurses' Database).

gentrification of nursing, 40 per cent of St George's recruits came from Classes III, IV and V.

Combining probationer analysis with data for other nursing ranks, it is clear that St George's (up to 1897, at least) was not selecting its nurses by class, but on perceived merit; and even further, that opportunities existed for women from lower social backgrounds to rise to positions of authority. Unlike St Thomas', King's, the London or UCH, St George's did not operate a class-based hierarchy within its Nursing Department. Unlike Jane Brook's findings, all social classes were afforded the same privileges and had similar opportunities for promotion. The findings from St George's support Maggs' argument that nursing became a social melting pot and that, regardless of a woman's class before entering the hospital, once there, she became first and foremost a nurse (1983).

Young and single or old and married?

A second characteristic of 'modern' nursing was the increasing presence of young, single women. This was illustrated well in the 'Sairey Gamp versus Nightingale Nurse' image published in the *Nursing Record* in 1888, portraying the 'new nurse' as smart, demure and young (*NR Supplement* 20 December 1888). Historians have asked whether this image reflected reality, or whether it was intended to project an aspiration for the new profession (Maggs 1980 and 1983; Summers 1989; Rafferty 1996; Bashford 1998).

A few studies have examined the change in age profile of nurse recruits in the Victorian period. In a review of nursing handbooks and advertisements in magazines, Maggs found the 'ideal' age for a nurse recruit to be between 25 and 35 (1980). However, the average age of probationers at the four hospitals in his study was lower than this advertised 'ideal', falling within the 21–25 age group (1980).

Several theories been proposed to explain the choice of 25 as the 'ideal' lower age limit. As both a physically and emotionally demanding job, nursing was not considered suitable for younger women. Contemporary scientific thinking agreed that women reached maturity (both physically and emotionally) in their mid-twenties, and to employ younger women in demanding roles would put their health at risk. Such women would also threaten the efficient running of the hospital, if they were not strong enough for the work (Abel-Smith 1960; Maggs 1983). The lower age limit also coincided with the age at which women were expected to be considering marriage, and therefore the choice of marriage or nursing would have to be made. If the age limit was set higher, there would be fewer women to choose from, but if it was set too low, women could be lost to marriage after only a few years service (Maggs 1983; Thompson 1988).[60]

A study of Birmingham General Hospital (based on census returns) has shown that the average age of nurses fell from 42 in 1841 to 27 in 1891.

There was also a significant change in nurses' marital status. In 1861 nearly 50 per cent of nurses were reported to be either married or widowed, but by 1891 all but one were single, this remaining nurse being a widow (Wildman 1999).

At St George's Hospital, the rules on age changed little over the period of study. In a published set of rules in 1836, the Matron was expected to be between 30 and 45 when recruited, and unmarried. Retirement was set at no later than 65. These rules changed in 1897 (on the departure of Mrs Coster) when the retirement age was reduced to 60. Restrictions on status were also clarified over time, being widened to include widows, providing they had no dependent children.

Similarly, age limits for regular nurses and probationers changed little: nurses and probationers should be between 25 and 40 on joining the hospital. The upper age limit was reduced to 30 in 1898, and some months later the lower limit was reduced to 23 (SGHCON/2, 10 March 1898). This reduction in the upper limit must have caused problems, as almost immediately it was raised again, to 35 (SGHCON/2, 8 May 1899).

Nurses and probationers were expected to be able to read, and by the 1890s, the ability to write was also required – although neither of these skills is mentioned in the rules. The new rules also introduced height restrictions (probationers should be between 5 feet 3 inches and 5 feet 6 inches in height), a move *The Hospital*, referred to as, 'A curious notice … attached to the regulations for Probationers' (SGHCON/2, 10 March 1898; *H/NM*, 3 October 1896: 5). Women who wore glasses were prohibited from entering the hospital under these same rules (SGHCON/2, 10 March 1898). The height restrictions were lifted some months later, replaced with a more general statement that probationers should be of average height and physique. The rule prohibiting the wearers of glasses from being admitted is odd and no evidence has been found of a similar restriction at other hospitals.

The average age of St George's nurses decreased from 39 in 1841 to 28 in 1901, mirroring Stuart Wildman's finding for the Birmingham Hospital (see Figure 2.8). While it was not unusual to find nurses over 40 working at St George's in the 1840s and 1850s, by the end of the century such women represented only a very small fraction of the workforce, reflecting the approximate numbers of head nurses employed – in 1891, when head nurses accounted for 18 per cent of the nursing department, nearly 20 per cent of nurses were over 35. The increasing youth of the Nursing Department reflects the growing number of probationers being recruited, and the emergence of probationers as the dominant group by the 1890s. By 1894, probationers accounted for 65 of the total staff of 120 and the fact that over 80 per cent of nurses were below 35 years of age in 1891 reflects this.

Although the trend towards youthful nurses was relentless, an analysis of age on commencement of employment (as opposed to age of nurses in the department at census years) indicates that the hospital was prepared

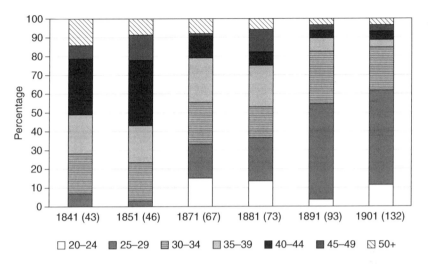

Figure 2.8 Age profile of nurses at St George's (source: St George's Nurses' Database).

to hire nurses at the top end of the age range. Up to the 1880s, at least 25 per cent of recruits were over 35 when they took up their positions (SGHNDB). But as the joint policies of internal promotion and increased numbers of probationers took hold, by the 1890s, all recruits were under 35 and only a few were over 30. The hospital was also prepared to bend its own rules on the lower age limit, particularly at times when it was difficult to maintain the Nursing Department at full strength, as in the 1870s.

The nationwide trend towards younger nurses became a topic of discussion in the nursing journals in the 1890s. Many older nurses complained that they were discriminated against in favour of younger colleagues, and this applied not just to those starting their careers, but to higher posts as well. One matron wrote to *The Hospital,*

> Candidates over 40 are entirely put on one side for younger and far less experienced ones. ... If a matron, sister or nurse is out of work at 45, what is to happen to her till she comes in for her pension at 60? She is not ill and cannot claim sick pay; but she is to be put out on one side for younger people.
>
> (*H/NM,* 1 June 1889: xxxiv)

The Hospital received many letters on this theme, often combined with complaints that lady nurses (who did not need to earn a living) were taking work from those who depended on it:

> When will it end? Is it just that ladies with large incomes ... who because of the restlessness of the age ... should rush into the nursing

world and take the bread from those less-favoured gentlewomen who
have no resource but to work for their living?

(*H/NM*, 8 June 1889: xxxviii)

The blame was laid at the door of economics: younger, less experienced
women could be paid less than their older counterparts; and ladies, whose
prime motivation was not financial, might agree to work for very low
wages, or even without payment at all (*H/NM*, 12 October 1889: ix). A
rather more flippant argument for preferring younger candidates was put
forward by the *Nursing Record*. It suggested that the governors of Peterbor-
ough Workhouse had selected an 'attractive young nurse' over an 'elderly
candidate' because her appearance 'might induce the Visiting Committee
to attend more regularly' (*NR*, 21 October 1893: 186).

The increasing youth of nurses at St George's illustrates the hospital's
rapidly growing dependence on probationers to provide patient care,
rather than positive discrimination against older nurses, per se. Not surprisingly, the change in age profile was also mirrored by a similar change
in marital status (see Figure 2.9).

By 1901, over 90 per cent of St George's nurses were single, in complete
contrast to the situation in 1851 when 70 per cent were either married or
widowed. The trend towards single nurses is similar to that found at Birmingham General Hospital, but appears to have started later at St
George's. In Wildman's study, single women represented 70 per cent of
the workforce by 1871, whereas in the same census, equal numbers of St
George's nurses were single, married or widowed (Wildman 1999;
SGHNDB).

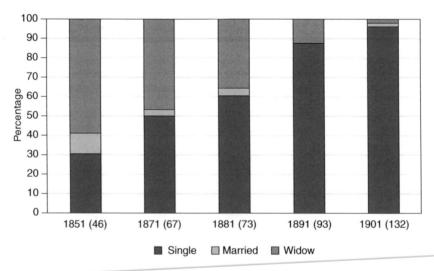

Figure 2.9 Marital status of nurses at St George's (source: Decennial censuses
1841–1901 (excluding 1861)).

St George's was very tolerant of its nurses' family situations, apparently willing to employ married women whose husbands were away from home, possibly in the military or, in at least one case, incarcerated in a lunatic asylum. It also employed women with young children. A list of questions on the probationers' application form, from 1871, supports this: those probationers who declared themselves widowed were asked how many children they had, and how they would be provided for (SGHCON/1, 28 November 1871).

Harriet Coster had three children under 12 on her appointment; and the records make mention of several nurses who left to return to their children.[61] In some cases, the hospital may have been unaware of the existence of such families, but in many it was known.[62] Sarah Wall, who joined the hospital in 1884 as a probationer, was dismissed when it transpired that she had four children. She had admitted to only one in her application, and it is likely that she was dismissed for lying on her application, rather than for having four children (SGHCON/1, 9 March 1885). As late as the 1880s, at least 40 per cent of the nurses were either married or widowed, and it is more than likely that a large number of them had at least one dependent child. The hospital must have been aware of this. However, as long the existence of children did not affect the efficient running of the hospital, it appears that mothers were accepted, especially at times when recruitment was hard.

Geographic origins

Where did St George's nurses come from: were they local women, or had they been drawn to London from the provinces? Stuart Wildman's Birmingham study found that, up to 1881, the majority of nurses was born in the immediate vicinity of the hospital, but by 1891, less than 50 per cent of nurses were born locally. Instead, most came from other areas of England, significantly, from Scotland, Wales and Ireland (Wildman 1999). At Leeds Infirmary, a high percentage came from the immediate rural surroundings; whereas Southampton tended to recruit from 'other urban areas', and at Portsmouth nurses came from within the city (Brooks 2001; Maggs 1980). The majority of nurse recruits to UCH were from English towns outside London, according to Janet Likeman. She found only a few from outside England (Likeman 2002).

The origins of St George's nurses were determined from place of birth data in the decennial censuses, and complemented by information on last known address before joining the hospital (from the hospital's Nurse Registers.). The data was analysed by date of start to determine if any migratory trends could be discerned (see Figure 2.10).

The analysis reveals that a significant number of St George's nurses did not originate from the immediate vicinity of the hospital, even in the early years of the study. In those early decades approximately 30 per cent of

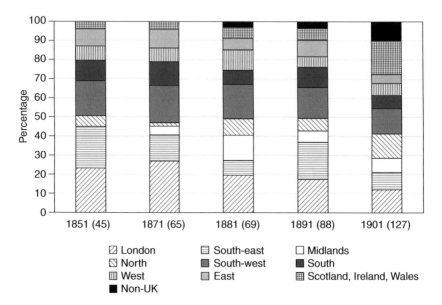

Figure 2.10 Place of birth of nurses at St George's (source: Decennial censuses 1851, 1871, 1881, 1891, 1901. South-east includes all counties surrounding London; Midlands (Derbyshire, Leicestershire, Northamptonshire, Nottinghamshire, Oxfordshire, Staffordshire, Warwickshire and Worcestershire); North (Durham, Northumberland, Yorkshire, Cheshire, Cumbria and Lancashire); South (Hampshire, Dorset, Sussex, Cornwall, Devon); West (Gloucestershire, Herefordshire, Shropshire, Somerset, Wiltshire); East (East Anglia, Cambridgeshire and Lincolnshire)).

nurses were born in London and a further 20 per cent came from counties adjacent to the capital.[63] However, by 1901, less than a quarter of recruits were local women: geographically they were diverse, arriving at the hospital from all corners of the United Kingdom and even further afield. Women from the north (in particular Yorkshire) and the south and west made up the largest group of English nurses (15 per cent), while 12 per cent came from Scotland. A growing number were born outside the British Isles, several in India, presumably the daughters of the colonial civil service.

St George's data appear to conform to generally accepted patterns of female migration during the nineteenth century. Saville has postulated that women were more migratory than men, and formed a pattern of migration from rural to urban areas, usually over short distances. He also found evidence of migration over much longer distances, if the move was towards 'great centres of commerce and industry' (quoted in Maggs 1983). According to F.M.L. Thompson, young unmarried girls 'poured into towns in their hundreds and thousands' in search of domestic service, coming from great distances and 'deeply rural' backgrounds (1988: 179). It is possible that some women made the same journey to take up nursing, but experience at St George's suggests that women left home as domestic servants and turned to nursing later. Many of the women born outside London had moved there prior to joining the hospital. Lack of data prohibits a statistical analysis of this phenomenon, but anecdotal evidence supports this. Alice Bradley, the widow of a Kent man (but born in Devon), had been a general servant in Westminster preceding her appointment in 1864 as nurse at the hospital; while Elizabeth Coleridge, also born in Devon, worked in London as a parlour maid for at least ten years before joining St George's in 1878 (SGHNDB).

Conclusion

In drawing together the various strands of this chapter, it can be concluded that the profile of a St George's nurse followed a trend which mirrored, to a certain extent, the 'ideal' nurse promoted by nurse reformers. As the century progressed, she became younger, less likely to be married and more likely to come from the higher classes in society. However, unlike most other London hospitals, St George's offered no special inducements to these higher-class women and appeared not to favour them unduly when considering candidates for promotion. There is no evidence to support Janet Likeman's thesis that by the end of the century nursing, here, was dominated by middle-class women. Neither does it support the argument that although all social classes were admitted, ordinary nurses and nurse managers were strictly segregated. There are some parallels, in terms of class, with Ann Simnet's data from Bart's (see Figure 2.1), where nurse recruits from all social classes were present in the 1880s, although by 1892 recruits at Bart's were derived exclusively from middle-class women, in complete contrast to the situation at St George's.

St George's Nursing Department, by the end of the century, appeared to conform most closely to Christopher Maggs' description of a 'melting pot' containing representatives from all strata in society. Once they joined the hospital, nurses entered a new hierarchy, one defined solely by skill and experience.

Change in social class was driven more by external factors than by a successful effort on the part of the hospital to attract 'ladies'; and the hospital may have benefited in this regard from the new fashionable status of nursing. By the late nineteenth century many more women from the higher social classes were looking for work as nurses, and St George's, perhaps because of its location in a very fashionable part of London, was an attractive proposition. The hospital professed a desire to attract a 'better class' of woman, and although some general steps were taken to facilitate this objective, it never instituted a scheme directly targeted at such women – unlike most of its competitor institutions. It seems more likely that by 'better class', the hospital was referring to the general demeanour and education of its nurse recruits, rather than to a specific social category. The lack of paying probationers may be explained by the hospital's brief, but unsuccessful, dalliance with lady nurses in the 1860s. It may have feared that paying probationers would feel entitled (by dint of having paid fees) to make demands regarding their conditions of employment and accommodation. Perhaps, they were just more trouble than they were worth, their contribution to the hospital finances not deemed sufficient compensation. Equally, as there appeared to be little trouble attracting such women to join as regular probationers, a paying probationer scheme may have appeared unnecessary.

The other striking feature of St George's in comparison with other hospitals is its attitude to promotion. For most of the period under review, women at St George's were promoted to head nurse based on ability and experience, rather than their social class. Mrs Coster had benefited herself from such egalitarian views, and may have influenced this policy. The arrival of Florence Smedley (a 'new' nurse, formally trained at Bart's) seems to herald a change, and by the end of the century class appeared to have had more bearing on promotion.

The increasing youth of recruits occurred as a direct result of decisions to staff the hospital predominantly with probationers, who by definition were under 30 years of age. As the proportion of probationers increased, so the average age of nurses decreased. Equally, as internal promotion policies reduced recruits from outside, the number of married and widowed nurses fell to almost zero by the end of the century. This is unlikely to have been as a result of discrimination against married or widowed women, but rather a logical outcome of a policy which recruited young, unmarried probationers, who then went on to fill more senior roles as they became vacant.

This analysis reveals a much more complex picture regarding the profile of late-Victorian nurses than might be imagined from contemporary reports. A study of the nineteenth century Nurse Register for Sydney Hospital in Australia, by historian Judith Godden, has revealed similar results. As Godden concluded: 'Nurse probationers [at Sydney Hospital] are far from the mythical, middle-class, air-brushed angels of the Nightingale nursing myth' (2003: 38). The more detailed studies that are carried out on the composition of actual nineteenth-century nursing departments, the further the orthodox view nursing in this period is thrown into doubt.

Pen Portrait 2 Eliza Ockenden – three generations of night nurses

Eliza Ockenden's career at St George's was brief. She joined as a night nurse in April 1883, but left 19 months later, in ill health. She was only 33. There was a constant and underlying grumble of sickness among the nurses. In the year Eliza left sickness levels had been unusually high. She was probably suffering from the first throes of the deadly scourge, tuberculosis. Six years later she was dead, phthisis the cause. Her friends wrote a letter to *The Hospital*, in which they criticized the Matron of St George's for not acknowledging her death.

Unlike earlier times, night nurses like Eliza were trained women, trusted with the care of their patients, almost unsupervised. Life as a night nurse was unremitting. There was no respite from the antisocial hours. Work started at 9.30 p.m. and finished at 9.30 a.m., with no breaks: 'tea' and 'supper' were taken on the wards. It was a lonely existence.

Eliza witnessed the scandal of her manager, Night Superintendent Hope, being 'asked to leave', accused of spreading malicious stories about nurses. The incident must have enlivened the dead hours of the night nurses' duty, and been the subject of much whispering amongst them in dark corners of their wards.

Eliza's nursing career had followed a familiar pattern. She trained at the Middlesex, worked for a while as a private nurse, before joining St George's. Nursing and St George's were in her blood. Both her mother and grandmother had been night nurses at the hospital. Margaret Ockenden, her grandmother, had worked when night nurses were mere 'watchers', rather than trained carers. The great revolution in night nursing (when experienced nurses replaced the likes of Margaret) saw her demoted to the role of 'cleaner'. Times were different then. Margaret lived at home, going to the hospital each night to work. She did this night in, night out for 18 years, finally retiring on a pension of eight shillings a week, in recognition of her long and dedicated service. Eliza's mother was probably encouraged to take up the work by her mother-in-law. The family lived close to the hospital, and it would have been convenient. By 1871, the family's ties to St George's were further strengthened. Both Eliza's father and younger brother were recorded in the census as anatomical porters. Given their close proximity to the hospital, and the family's previous connections, it seems plausible that father and son had joined the 'family firm'. By 1881, Eliza's father had been promoted to pathological sub-curator.

Eliza's story illustrates several important themes: the role of family in influencing choice of occupation; the importance of the hospital to the neighbourhood economy; and the hidden impact of tuberculosis on working people's lives.

There was no mention of TB in Eliza's hospital records, but her death certificate states it plainly; and the anger of her friends that the Matron refused to acknowledge her death suggests this was a disease to which no one wanted to admit.

3 Probationer schemes

Education or cheap labour?

The introduction of systematic nurse training was as much a part of nineteenth-century reform of the profession as changes in class and age profile discussed in the previous chapter. In traditional histories, Nightingale is credited with this innovation but, as with many such claims, this is now questioned. As Monica Baly and Carol Helmstader have argued, her contribution to nurse training represented a continuum of a process which began with nursing sisterhoods, rather than a revolution (Baly 1987; Helmstadter 1996).

Whoever was responsible, it is indisputable that nurse training became longer and increasingly sophisticated as the century progressed. Originally an informal arrangement, whereby women acquired their skills through experience on the wards, by the end of the century nurse education had metamorphosed into a structured three-year course of theoretical and practical study.

Advances in medicine, particularly its emergence as a more scientific discipline, created an evolutionary pressure on the role of the nurse. From being little more than simple carers with a main responsibility to keep patients comfortable, nurses were increasingly expected to perform technical interventions (Helmstadter 2002). Such changes brought benefits to nurse leaders and doctors alike. For nurse reformers, the technical nature of 'new nursing' offered the opportunity to define a body of knowledge, which could be used to redefine nursing as a profession rather than a quasi-domestic service occupation (Simonton 2001). For doctors, the availability of better educated nurses created opportunities for delegation of their more routine (or mundane) tasks.

However, advances in medical science do not provide the only explanation for the emergence of formal nurse training. Pressures in Victorian society also contributed to the phenomenon: not least the 'surplus women problem', and a new interest in education for young middle-class women. Improved nurse training, it was argued, would attract such women – who were entering the workplace for the first time in significant numbers – by offering an opportunity for further study. At the other end of the social scale, it also resonated with Victorian society's obsession with controlling and moulding the lower classes. Laden with middle-class ideals of morality and character, nurse training would instil such values in lower-class recruits (Dean and Bolton 1980).

This chapter explores the impact of these social pressures on the development of nurse training, specifically from the perspectives of the main protagonists: the nurses, the medical men and the hospital managers.

Nurse reformers and nurse education

The nursing sisterhoods of the 1840s took in women of mixed social class to train as nurses: lower-class women to work on the wards, higher-class women to be nurse managers (Baly 1987; Dingwall *et al.* 1988). St John's House was one of several such Anglican sisterhoods to emerge in the mid-nineteenth century (Bradshaw 2000; Moore 1988).

Reflections of the St John's House ethos can be seen in Nightingale's school. The distinction between ladies and regular nurses (in terms of their financial arrangements with the institution), the insistence that sisters trained with the regular nurses and the class basis of role assignment were all features of both institutions (Moore 1988). Nightingale, it is said, was attracted by the sisterhoods' focus on the development of character and instillation of discipline (Bradshaw 2000). Recent work by Irish historians has tentatively suggested reflections of the Catholic Sisters of Mercy – whom Nightingale encountered in the Crimea – in her plans for St Thomas'. This model, referred to as 'careful nursing', combined physical and emotional care of the sick, with a spiritual perspective. Among its tenets were 'creation of a restorative environment ... perfect skill in fostering safety and comfort ... and health education', elements which can all be located within Nightingale's own philosophy of nursing (Meehan 2003). The origins of Nightingale's insistence that nurses should 'nurse the room' are clearly visible in 'careful nursing', as is her belief that the job of nursing was to create an environment in which the body was able to heal itself (Gamarnikow 1978). The inclusion of hygiene, sanitation and an element of psychology into Nightingale's ideas for nurse education indicates she was interested in more than just the moral character of her nurses (Baly 1986 [1997]).[1]

Nightingale broke from the sisterhood model in one important aspect: her nurses did not take religious vows. Her experiences in the Crimea revealed the potential for conflicts of loyalty if nurses served two masters; she also suspected that nursing sisters placed undue focus on spiritual healing at the expense of physical healing. Reflecting these concerns, her plan for a nurse training school required applicants to be committed Christians, but stopped short of establishing a new religious order (Holcombe 1973; Vicinus 1985).

The ability of sisterhoods to attract recruits has been attributed, in part at least, to the need to create employment for single, middle- and upper-class women, although this is not to deny the religious influence, already discussed in Chapter 1. Nurse reformers hoped to appeal to this same demographic and adopted elements of the sisterhoods' approach to help them achieve this, including the provision of more formal education and training (Maggs 1983).[2] Furthermore, if the completion of training was recognized, either through the award of a certificate or, even more enticingly by the opportunity for promotion to a position of authority, the attractiveness of nursing could be enhanced (Maggs 1983). Thus, hospitals and nurse reformers hoped that by incorporating such elements into their nurse training schemes, respectable women would be persuaded to overlook the obvious disadvantages of nursing work – the potential loss of status (during training at least), the squalid conditions and the laborious nature of the work (Maggs 1983).

In mid-century, the idea of training women for work was controversial. While training with regard to one's position in society was widespread (as the plethora of Victorian etiquette manuals testifies), there was little in the way of formal education for young women, or training of women (of any class) for work (Johnson 1970; Langland 1995). Respectable middle-class women did not work, but were trained at their mothers' sides to be wives and mothers themselves: working-class women were considered untrainable (Rose 1992; Simonton 2001). Further, the perceived inevitability of marriage rendered the training of women both unnecessary and wasteful (Burman 1979). Training and education was heavily gendered. While male activities were regarded as skills, to be acquired, honed and refreshed through training, female activities were regarded as an inherent part of their femaleness, not skills at all (Simonton 2001). Following this argument, woman's supposed natural ability to care for the sick, therefore, negated any need to provide specific training for nurses.

Other female occupations received similar treatment. Female seamstresses, for instance, were usually considered unskilled, as sewing was a natural talent acquired from their mothers. Male tailors, on the other hand, underwent long apprenticeships and were regarded as a highly skilled workforce (John 1986; Rose 1992).[3]

So to train nurses was wasteful: women were natural carers requiring no specialist skills. Nursing's close association with domestic service also predicated against training and lowered its appeal to middle-class women. These entrenched positions had to be overturned if nurse reformers were to achieve their goals. Catherine Wood (Matron at the Hospital for Sick Children (HSC) and a strong proponent of nurse education) agreed that women possessed natural traits making them ideal carers, but argued that to be efficient nurses they needed training in the best way to use these talents. 'Many [women]', she wrote, 'have the will to tend the sick, but few have the skill to do it' (Wood 1888).[4] In constructing such arguments, reformers sought to draw clear distinctions between nursing and domestic service, which up to this point were in danger of being seen as two sides of the same coin.

The 'surplus women' problem stimulated a new interest in the education and training of young middle-class women. In the 1850s, institutions such as Queen's and Bedford Colleges began training women to be teachers, while the Society for Promoting Employment for Women offered courses in a range of occupations. A decade later, female medical colleges were beginning to emerge, and the first colleges for women were founded at Oxford and Cambridge (Gleadle 2001; Steinbach 2004).[5]

Against this background, the first nurse training schools were posited. Taking their lead from Queen's, the new nursing schools provided opportunities for respectable women who needed to earn their living. The offer of training which combined theoretical and practical elements helped to distinguish nursing from domestic service and provided a realistic alternative to teaching. The strategy was ultimately successful: by the end of the century respectable young women were flocking to nursing. Evidence that they saw it as a positive alternative to other forms of further education abounds in the letters pages of newspapers, as this example – from the mother of a nurse – demonstrates:

> Just now [nursing] is the fashion for those who do not care to go to Girton ... and who find staying at home to help the mother is out of date. Not very long ago, to rush into a Sisterhood, if not to become a nun, was the panacea for all home trials. Now to be a nurse takes the lead.
>
> (*The Standard*, 9 March 1889: 2)

Nursing had become fashionable. For some, it was never more than a flirtation, as the quote above suggests, but for others it not only provided a form of further education, but promised a career with opportunities for advancement.

While new middle-class recruits may have been attracted by the promise of education, nurse leaders had additional considerations in deciding the content of their training schemes. Hospitals were potentially dangerous places for young middle-class women, where all social classes and both sexes were thrown into close contact (Vicinus 1985). In this atmosphere of social chaos, strict and complex rules were needed to define relationships and behaviour (Gamarnikow 1978; Rafferty 1996; Judd 1998). As Victorian society was defined by a complex etiquette, so too was nursing: manuals for trainees provided instruction on nursing procedures, but also included chapters on 'hospital etiquette'.[6] Nurse training, therefore, was as much about building character, reinforcing moral strength and instilling discipline, as about acquiring nursing skills and medical knowledge. In fact, training focused to such an extent on character building as to suggest that most recruits, far from being respectable middle-class women, were in fact from the working classes, and in dire need of reshaping into the image of their middle-class sisters.

From its inception, the training school at St Thomas' included lectures on elementary sciences for all nurses, while more advanced lectures were restricted to lady probationers. The distinction was partly driven by differing levels of prior education between the two groups, which made it impossible to teach them together; but was also probably connected to the different roles they were expected to assume (Bradshaw 2000). There is also a suggestion that the lady probationers gained access to this higher level of education because they demanded it. The enhanced curriculum was criticized by St Thomas' medical faculty, who accused the lecturer of producing ancillary doctors rather than nurses; Nightingale was also sceptical, believing that nursing and medicine should complement, not replicate, skills and knowledge (Baly 1987). The power of fashion (as evinced by the oversubscription for places) proved irresistible, and as other training schemes began to include a theoretical element, any attempt to remove or curtail such content from the St Thomas' scheme would have appeared a retrograde step (Baly 1987).

The balance between theoretical and moral training became a defining issue in the battle which was emerging between the pro- and anti-registration factions in the nursing world. Ethel Fenwick and her pro-registration colleagues modelled their ideas for nurse training on the medical curriculum, combining a significant element of theoretical teaching with prolonged practical experience, prior to qualification and formal entry into the profession (McGann 1992; Weir 2000). Anti-registrationists, such as Eva Luckes (with Nightingale in the background), decried the focus on theory, claiming an overemphasis on theoretical knowledge would detract from character training, essential for the formation of a good nurse (Rafferty 1996; Bradshaw 2000).

The views of Catherine Wood demonstrate the fine nuances in the arguments about education. While she strongly supported a sound theoretical element in the education of nurses, she also emphasized the importance of character development. 'Deft hands, the quiet manner, the power of sympathy, the adaptability, the gentle patience, the firmness and steadiness of purpose, and above all the grand unselfishness', were all traits which nurse education had to develop in a trainee nurse (Wood 1894: 54). Like Nightingale and Luckes, she was concerned that an overemphasis on theoretical education would lead nurses to forget their natural role. Criticizing the 'fashion' for putting theory above moral teaching, she wrote, 'Small blame to a nurse ... [if] having her rank determined by her proficiency in theory, she forgets that she is not the doctor' (Wood 1897).

Wood's concern that an overemphasis on medical subjects would lead nurses to think themselves equal to doctors was a common theme and was one of the chief arguments against including such material in the curriculum. Doctors cited it frequently, exposing their own insecurities that educated nurses might question their authority and even compete against them for business. Even nurse leaders who supported better education for nurses were very aware of its dangers, and wary of denting the fragile egos of the medical profession. While speaking volubly on the subject of nursing as an independent profession, in private they seemed unable to envisage a way of achieving their goals without the support of doctors.

One of the problems in defining an appropriate course of nurse training stemmed from a lack of agreement on the nature of nursing itself. In 1859, Nightingale wrote that, 'the elements of nursing are all but unknown' and the debates and disagreements on nurse education, training and professionalization, which dominated the following 50 years, arose, in part, as an attempt to resolve Nightingale's conundrum. (Nightingale 1861: 15). Nursing was either a 'moral metier' (as espoused by Nightingale and her followers) or a profession founded on science, as Fenwick would have it (Rafferty 1996). But the problem faced by Fenwick and her supporters was the absence of a coherent but unique knowledge base on which a unique scientific nursing curriculum could be built. Nurse leaders had no choice but to borrow directly from the medical curriculum and in so doing handed control over the content of training to doctors. In the process, nurses' claims to autonomy were irrevocably damaged (Weir 2000).[7]

In the early years of reform, nurses attempted to define a niche for themselves by stressing the importance of hygiene and sanitary care of the sick (Garmanikow 1978; Vicinus 1985). Being primarily concerned with cleanliness and good household management, both fell naturally within women's remit (Bashford 1998). But nurses failed to capitalize on this one of area of knowledge they could have made their own. Changing attitudes to cleaning work, and the conflation of hygiene and sanitary work with domestic chores, probably made such a move unattractive; and lady nurses more used to supervising cleaning than doing it themselves, saw to it that hygiene was relegated to the level of scrubbers and ward maids. The role of nurse-hygienist survived to a limited extent in district and private nursing; but the main body of nursing, in thrall to the new medical science, confined itself to administering and supervising medical care (Gamarnikow 1978).

Thus one plank of Nightingale's definition of nursing – that nurses should 'nurse the room' – was surrendered and an opportunity to define an area of healthcare and a body of knowledge which nurses could claim as their own was lost (Gamarnikow 1978). The failure to retain ownership of hygiene in the sick room has resonances even today, amid the scandals of dirty hospitals, outsourced cleaning contracts, and the connection to a rising incidence of hospital-acquired infection.

The appropriation of hygiene into a body of nursing knowledge was also impeded by other developments. As theories of disease became increasingly scientific, the spiritual element of hygiene and sanitation (which Nightingale had invoked through her adherence to the miasmatic theory of disease) diminished, transforming them from quasi-spiritual (female) subjects into pure (male) sciences (Rafferty 1996; Bashford

1998).[8] Women's claim to be the natural keepers of the knowledge was, thereby, eroded and hygiene and sanitation were absorbed into the body of general medical science (Vicinus 1985). Why nurse leaders allowed this to occur requires further study, by asking questions regarding the gendered nature of science and the close links between hygiene and domestic work.

Having eschewed sanitation and hygiene, which could have helped to define a unique body of nursing knowledge, nurse reformers had little recourse but to adopt elements of the medical curriculum into their own training. This enabled them to attract middle-class women into the occupation, but at the great cost of damaging their claim to be a profession independent of medicine.

Doctors and nurse education

Nightingale's focus on the development of character and obedience in hospital nurses – at the expense of medical knowledge – played to the egos of the medical men. In the mid-nineteenth century, the fragile monopoly of the medical profession was threatened by several competing groups, among which the domiciliary nurses loomed large (Summers 1989). Such women, often working independently of doctors, operated within their own network of contacts, charging lower fees and competing for custom (Summers 1989; Rafferty 1995). Thus, when hospitals became the focus for nurse training – bringing it under the close scrutiny of doctors – the move played directly into doctors' hands (Bashford 1998). It enabled them to ration nurses' access to knowledge, and to dictate the nature of the relationship between doctor and nurse (Gamarnikow 1978). The professionalization debate was never about raising the position of nurses within the medical hierarchy, but was, instead, about establishing a role for nursing within an uncontested hierarchy which placed doctors at the very top (Gamarnikow 1978).

This subordinate role was further reinforced by nurse reformers' invocation of middle-class family structures to create safe spaces in hospitals where women could work (Gamarnikow 1978). Doctors were the 'fathers' of the institutions and naturally assumed a patriarchal relationship towards the nurses. From this position, they were able to dictate the rules under which nurses would live and work. Equally, nurses (in behaviour ingrained by family experience) were expected to accept doctors' orders and teachings without question (Gamarnikow 1978). However, the existence of complex rules for nurses, and the intense focus on discipline and obedience, suggest that the transition from home into hospital was never completely achieved. If it had been, surely such focus would have been unnecessary (Bashford 1998).

That nurses found themselves in this subordinate position to doctors had major implications for the development of nurse training. A probationer's life was regulated at every turn, dictated by myriad rules controlling her day in minute detail. Rules defined how she should relate to patients, other nurses and, most importantly, to doctors and hospital managers (Bashford 1998). According to Bashford, this combination of rigid regulations and behavioural training was designed to produce Foucault's 'docile bodies' which would 'operate as one wishes, with the techniques, the speed and the efficiency that one determines' (Bashford 1998; Foucault 1991: 138). Nurses, thus trained, would be a valuable aid to doctors, but completely devoid of threat to the medics' professional status. They would form an efficient workforce, without necessarily understanding, working almost from reflex (Bashford 1998). Neither Nightingale nor Wood agreed with this definition of the role, believing nurses should not work blindly but with 'intelligent obedience'. Nevertheless, they were entirely in agreement that a nurse's natural position was subordinate to the medical profession (Nightingale 1861 [1952]: 131).[9]

The choice of hospitals as the primary location for nurse training was not inevitable. Independent colleges, along the lines of teaching colleges such as Queen's, could have been established for nurse training. Nurse leaders could have adopted an apprenticeship approach, assigning trainees to working nurses in the community, to learn by observation and experience. Instead, hospital-based training schools became the norm, tied inextricably to their father-institutions: the result of doctors' determination to seize control of the 'new nursing'.

Hospitals did make logical training grounds: they offered a wide variety of patient-types from which trainee nurses could learn, and provided a controlled environment in which behaviour could be monitored and practice constrained. The opportunity to mould nursing staff to their own requirements took on increasing importance for doctors as the century progressed and hospitals developed into centres of medical knowledge, as opposed to simple warehouses for the sick. They were transforming into large laboratories where patients and diseases could be observed and data gathered.[10]

As subjects in a museum of disease, patients needed careful observation and those observations had to be minutely recorded. This was not a practical use of doctors' time, which was divided between work at the hospital and more lucrative private practice. A trustworthy surrogate was needed, and this was the role envisaged for the trained nurse. Such duties could have been handed to an increased number of medical dressers, but too many doctors in training posed a serious threat to professional stability (Rafferty 1996; Allen 2001).[11] The alternative was to create a new type of assistant, reliable and trustworthy but without threat to the integrity of the medical profession. The reformed nurse fit the bill perfectly, and by locating their training in hospitals, doctors could ensure that the new nurse was schooled to meet these needs. Mindful of the threat that educated nurses might pose to their fragile authority, doctors were also quick to reinforce the subordinate position of nursing. Training, therefore, was designed to instil a keen sense of observation, tempered by a strict adherence to doctors' orders.

Medical men were split over the issue of nurse education. Some saw the benefit of well-trained, knowledgeable nurses assisting them in their work. With some medical training, nurses could become accurate and reliable observers and recorders of a patient's condition, transforming them into the eyes and ears of the doctor in his absence. As one doctor wrote in 1873:

> Her knowledge of anatomy, physiology, pathology and the action of drugs should be thorough, though not necessarily very minute.... She should also understand the value and meaning of symptoms.... She should be able to record ... pulse and thermometer, and know how to act in an emergency in the absence of a doctor.... They must [be admitted to] lectures ... so that in their sphere they be no automatic servants of, but rational fellow-workers with, the physician.
>
> (Editorial, *BMJ*, 4 January 1873 quoted in Gamarnikow 1991: 113)

Even this doctor, who clearly supported the education of nurses, was careful to define the boundaries of the role. A nurse should be educated, but not in 'minute and extensive' detail; and although she may be a 'rational fellow-worker' her 'sphere' of influence is decidedly different from that of the doctor.

For every doctor who supported nurse education, there were others who opposed it. Arguments against were often borrowed from the general debate on education for women, founded on social Darwinist interpretations of contemporary scientific developments (Burstyn 1980; McDermid 1995). Such arguments posited that, having smaller brains, women were less able to withstand sustained intellectual endeavour. Over-education led to excessive stimulation of the brain, which in turn resulted in nervous collapse and brain damage. Even more importantly, in Victorian eyes, such mental exertion could result in reproductive problems, rendering the woman incapable of performing the primary function for which she was created (Perkin 1993; Steinbach 2004).[12]

According to Gamarnikow, doctors used such arguments against nurse education to camouflage real concerns that the educated nurse posed a threat to their authority (Gamarnikow 1978). The medical profession had only recently secured its monopoly over healthcare, with state recognition of that status, and still exhibited symptoms of insecurity and paranoia (Parry and Parry 1976).[13] Educated nurses, if perceived as quasi-medical practitioners, would pose a threat to the medical profession. The following, from a doctor during the 1904 debate on nurse registration, shows the depth of feeling (and incredibly long institutional memory) within the profession:

When the Society of Apothecaries was established in the reign of King James I, it was laid down that [they were not] to attend people in disease ... [but] when they went round in times of epidemics ... they came to be asked about illness, and so they gradually came into practice. ... Exactly the same thing would happen with regard to nurses.

(House of Commons Select Committee on Registration of Nurses 1904, quoted in Ganarnikow 1978: 105)

Doctors who shared such fears believed nurses' access to the body of medical knowledge (by which the profession defined itself) should be kept to a necessary minimum. Dr West, founder of the HSC, encouraged limited education of nurses; he wanted them to exercise judgement in care, based on knowledge, but he also warned against overstepping the mark. In his handbook for children's nurses, he cautioned:

I must remind you that the nurse is not the doctor; that she never can be; that if she forgets her proper place, and tries to interfere with his duties, or to set herself above his directions, instead of being a blessing she will be a curse.

(West 1854: 16)

Dr Octavius Sturges, physician to the Westminster Hospital and the HSC, issued a similar caution to the Royal British Nursing Association (RBNA). He warned of the dangers to hospital discipline of nurses knowing too much, reminding them that 'like the soldier, [a nurse's] ruling characteristic should be obedience' (quoted in Anon. 1891: 53).

Sturges' concerns were common among doctors, and frequently aired in the pages of medical journals and daily papers. As one wrote in *The Lancet*,

To give nurses instruction as to the reason why ... this or that expedient [is] necessary would be to lift them ... out of their proper sphere, to demand for them complete education as medical practitioners and to transform them from nurses into doctors.

(*The Lancet*, 8 July,1876: 71)

Although these developments caused some alarm, the outcome was very much to the doctors' advantage. With training based on the medical curriculum, doctors could take a central, controlling position in nurse education. They ensured that lectures were restricted to areas of medical science *they* deemed appropriate for nurses; and also insinuated frequent reference to the nurses' duty of obedience to the medical profession. Nurse leaders acquiesced in this. If Nightingale had been uncertain as to what constituted nursing in 1859, by 1882 she had formulated a clearer picture:

> [Nurse] training is [designed to] teach a nurse to know her business ... to observe exactly, to understand, to know exactly, to tell exactly. ... Training has to make her, not servile, but loyal to medical orders and authorities. ... Training is to teach the nurse to handle the agencies within our control ... in strict obedience to the physician's or surgeon's power and knowledge.
>
> (quoted in Gamarnikow 1978: 107)

Improved education for nurses brought other benefits to doctors, besides producing 'docile bodies'. Not only could they be relied on to make accurate and regular observations of patients, but tasks considered routine and mundane by medical staff could be transferred to these new assistants (Weir 2000).

In a paper delivered in 1889, Dr Sturges – who, two years later, warned nurses against 'knowing too much' – praised them for their ability to carry out regular recordings of temperature:

> [Taking temperatures] is now left ... completely in her hands. It is a work of which she never tires. Six times, twelve times a day, even 24 times ... is the thermometer applied. If [this] were done by men I think we would hear more of the trouble and weariness of it.
>
> (Sturges 1889: 198)

In Sturges' view, the female characteristic of patience and attention to detail made her the ideal candidate for the job. Or, put another way, her lesser intellect prevented her from becoming overwhelmed with boredom by such repetitive tasks.[14] The delegation of such tasks would not only relieve doctors of their tedium or inconvenience, but (perhaps as importantly) would create additional time for doctors to devote to more challenging (or lucrative) aspects of medicine.

Returning to Dr Sturges, he also praised the nurse's ability to take the pulse but warned against any attempt to assess its character. Interpreting the pulse's strength, tension or length was part of the diagnostic process, and diagnosis was not the nurse's responsibility, under any circumstance (Sturges 1889). As Gamarnikow has said, nursing could be defined as observing and recording, and administering treatment and care, but interpretation of observations and the important decision as to who was, and was not, a patient were outside her 'sphere'. Diagnosis was sacrosanct to medicine (Gamarnikow 1978).

Post-operative patient management is another example of a once-medical task being transferred to nurses. Previously the domain of junior doctors or dressers, it involved close observation and regular refreshment of dressings. But as operations became more frequent and routine – with the advent of anaesthesia and better pain control – this also passed over to nurses. Operations such as tracheotomy and ovariotomy became commonplace and after-care of these patients fell to nurses.[15] Doctors, it seems, were experiencing some important advantages from the presence of trained nurses in hospitals, not least the ability to delegate to them routine work they had previously undertaken themselves.

To be an effective nurse, then, most doctors agreed that a certain level of medical knowledge was an advantage. There was less agreement on the ideal balance between moral and scientific content of training, but total agreement on the nurse's position with regard to her medical colleagues. This was always a subordinate one, regardless of the level of education attained (Williams 1980).

Hospital managers and nurse education

Reformers, therefore, had to battle against general prejudices against women's education, the protectionism of doctors, and the inertia of hospital matrons who had been in post for many years. They also had to convince a very sceptical group of men whose backgrounds were often in the world of business – the men who controlled the hospital finances. Without their support, attempts to improve nurse education would be problematic, and they may not have been easy to convince. The long delay between the Nightingale School opening (in 1860) and the introduction of nurse training schemes at other London hospitals (in the 1870s and 1880s) could be evidence of this scepticism.[16] A critical factor for any hospital administrator considering proposals to modernize his nursing department would be the fear of spiralling costs. At St Thomas' this concern was of secondary importance, as the school was supported by the Nightingale Fund, but at other hospitals increases in expenditure would have to be found from existing funds.[17]

However, on the positive side, probationers could make a positive financial contribution, and this opportunity would not go unnoticed by hospital administrators. Probationer schemes resembled apprenticeships; trainee nurses spent most of their time on the wards where learning and work were combined. Although most received a wage, it was much lower than that paid to established nurses and, consequently, substantial savings could be made if probationers were used in place of trained staff.[18] As nurse training courses became longer, the potential for cost savings grew. Early training courses lasted only one year, but by the end of the century, most schemes extended to three years.

Ethel Fenwick was one of the first to introduce a three-year scheme, when she was appointed Matron at Bart's in 1881. A pioneer of nurse education, she believed the extended period was essential to equip young nurses for the work (McGann 1992). Hospital administrators, on the other hand, saw extended training as an opportunity to further reduce labour costs. Although second- and third-year probationers received higher wages, they were still paid less than trained nurses, even though they worked full time on the wards. By the late nineteenth century the effect of these policies can be seen in the ratio of probationers to qualified nurses working at various hospitals. At the London there were four probationers to every staff nurse, while at Bart's the ratio was three to one (Helmstadter 1996). At St George's the probationer to staff nurse ratio was also four to one by the century's end, compared to one probationer to 2.5 ward nurses in the 1870s (SGHNDB). As already discussed in Chapter 2, by 1900, ward nursing was almost entirely in the hands of trainees in London hospitals.

Saving money on nursing bills was not the only financial incentive. Nurse training also offered enterprising hospitals an income-generating opportunity, by opening the schemes to women prepared to pay for the privilege. Most grasped the chance. The fees were consistent across London hospitals, at one guinea a week or 13 guineas a quarter, and for some hospitals it became an important revenue stream (see Appendix 2).[19] The HSC ran a very successful paying probationer scheme, which contributed (on average) 6 per cent to annual income, by the end of the century (HSC Archive).

By the 1890s, women were queuing up to enrol in nurse training schemes; and the inclusion of lectures in medical sciences was attracting better educated and more aspirational women into the occupation and the hospitals, improving the public perception of both.

But, as already suggested, this state of affairs did not come into being overnight or without pain. The quality and length of probationers' education differed wildly from school to school (there were no centrally agreed or administered standards) and individual hospitals were free to set up their own programmes. The rest of this chapter will focus on the development at St George's Hospital, and how the complex negotiations between the various interested parties were managed.

Nurse training at St George's

From the 1840s on, St George's Weekly Board returned repeatedly to the question of its Nursing Department and how to improve it. The hospital was already a large institution, with 350 beds, employing a matron and a staff of over 40 nurses. Nurses were organized by ward, each with a head nurse and several assistants. A separate group of nurses undertook night duty, managed by a Night Superintendent. The night nurses and assistant nurses were little more than servants: the bulk of the nursing duties being carried out by the head nurses, a group of very experienced women. In 1853, for instance, seven of the hospital's 16 head nurses had served over ten years in the role (SGHNDB). Whatever training assistant nurses required was gained from working alongside these very experienced women.

Formal nurse training at St George's was first discussed in the mid-1860s, in the aftermath of the failed attempt to turn nursing over to the sisters of St Peter's House.[20] Poor discipline among the assistant nurses was rife and it was hoped that a formal training scheme might attract a 'better class' of woman, whose superior standards of behaviour would rub off on the existing staff (SGHWB/33, 20 April 1866). In 1867, a committee appointed to look into the matter made a series of proposals: a maximum of seven women should be admitted as trainee nurses; they would be distributed throughout the wards under the direction of the Apothecary (not the Matron); and when considered to be sufficiently competent (no fixed period was defined) they would be employed officially as assistant nurses. The probationers, who should 'be able to read, write and read writing [*sic*]', be in good health and have a good character, must sign up for two years. In return they would receive £12 a year, with board and lodging (SGHWB/34, 22 May 1867). No women were actually employed under this scheme, as far as the records show.

The Matron's peripheral role in the supervision of probationers illustrates the nature of that post at the time: she was essentially a housekeeper, responsible for discipline among nurses but not for standards of nursing in the hospital. The Weekly Board identified this as one of the key obstacles to improving nursing standards and, in 1868, resolved to redefine it. The new Matron would take control of all aspects of the Nursing Department, and the role would be filled by a woman who had, 'practical experience of hospital nursing' (SGHWB/34, 29 January 1868). Furthermore, this woman would be of higher social standing than previous matrons, and reflecting this, the post would be renamed Lady Superintendent. The new rules for the Lady Superintendent (who quickly became known as Superintendent of Nurses, as already discussed in Chapter 2) included responsibility for the 'proper performance of the nurses, their moral conduct' and their attendance at weekly chapel (SGHWB/34, 1 April 1868).

Zepharina Veitch, appointed Lady Superintendent in 1869, was tasked with recruiting the first group of probationers. Within weeks of her appointment, she had 'four young women' ready to take up their places as probationers in the hospital (SGHCON/1, 22 March 1869).[21]

Three of these women have been identified. Anna Fice, Sarah Layton and Sarah Rudd all joined the hospital as probationers in April 1870. Only one can be said to address the hospital's desire to significantly improve the quality of recruits: Fice was the widow of a Wesleyan Minister – and therefore a very respectable member of society. Sadly, she died from blood poisoning within five months of being employed (SGHNR/1 Fice).

The other two women differed little from regular recruits, with the exception that they had no previous nursing experience. Sarah Layton (whose father was a journeyman carpenter and mother a laundress) had previously worked as a housemaid. She was almost dismissed at Christmas 1870 – after it was discovered she planned to marry in secret and continue working at the hospital – but was reprieved when an outbreak of smallpox needed all hands which could be mustered. She eventually left six months later to get married (SGHNR/1 Layton; SGHCON/1 19 December 1870).

Sarah Rudd was the most successful of these first three probationers. The daughter of a postmaster, she had worked as a lady's maid prior to joining St George's. She remained at the hospital for seven years, becoming head nurse in 1873. She finally resigned after a disagreement with the managers concerning new leave arrangements for assistant nurses, which she claimed left her short staffed. She probably also left nursing at this time: by 1881 she was unemployed and in 1891 was working as a laundress (SGHNR/1 Rudd; SGHCON/1, 22 August 1877; SGHNDB).

The introduction of a training scheme was expected to improve behaviour within the nursing body, not only by introducing a 'better class' of women into the hospital, but also by inculcating strict discipline at an early stage in a nurse's career. Historians have commented on the similarities between the organizational development of hospitals and that of factories, where managers believed it was necessary to break workers' spirit to mould a workforce of unquestioning obedience (Rafferty 1996). The benefits of training factory workers had already been demonstrated: according to Dr James Kay, such training taught the artisan 'the nature of his domestic and social relations … his political position in society and the moral and religious duties appropriate to it' (quoted in Johnson 1970: 102).[22] These were the very goals which the St George's governors had in mind: to train efficient nurses who knew their place in the hospital hierarchy, behaved in a sober and respectable manner, set a moral example to patients and demonstrated unswerving obedience.[23]

To give the training scheme an even greater chance of success, focus turned on recruits' previous experience. In the past, the hospital had preferred women with nursing experience, but when the probationer scheme was introduced, few recruits had such experience (see Figure 3.1). The hospital was obviously looking to a new pool of potential employees to fill probationer posts; primarily domestic servants, who represented 35 per cent of all such recruits. Furthermore, of the regular staff with previous nursing experience, the largest group (35 per cent) came from other major London hospitals, such as Bart's and Guy's. Clearly, previous policy had been to 'buy in' nursing experience, and it was the quality of this bought-in experience which was blamed for discipline problems within the department. Managers hoped that changes to recruitment policy, which favoured women with no preconceived ideas about nursing, would solve the discipline problems of previous years. Such women represented a blank canvas on which the hospital could stamp its own mark, ingraining its methods and standards of behaviour.

As the size of the probation department grew, so too did the percentage of recruits with previous nursing experience, thus the hospital was not eschewing entirely this qualification. It was not, however, generally

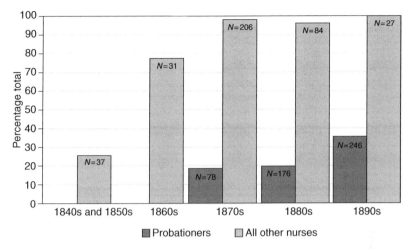

Figure 3.1 Previous nursing experience of nursing staff at St George's, 1840–1900 (source: St George's Nurses' Database constructed for this study from the following sources: Decennial censuses 1841, 1851, 1871, 1881, 1891 and St George's Nurse Registers and Minute Books 1850–1900. *N*=size of population. Figures for total nursing staff show percentage of all staff (including probationers) who had previous nursing experience).

obtained at the major London hospitals, but was more likely to have been received at a children's hospital, union infirmary or asylum (see Figure 3.2). Martha Vicinus has pointed out that, as a result of the minimum age limit at most large hospitals, women who wanted to train as nurses often worked in smaller institutions first to gain some experience. Children's and fever hospitals tended to take recruits at an earlier age – the work was often of a lighter and less complex nature – and they made ideal platforms for launching an embryonic nursing career (Vicinus 1985). Maggs has asserted (1983) that hospitals advised against gaining preliminary nursing experience at fever hospitals or asylums, for fear of acquiring 'bad habits' or 'partial training', but the St George's experience appears to contradict this. By the 1890s, nearly one quarter of probationers at St George's had worked in those unfavoured institutions.

The type of nursing experience which probationers brought to the hospital changed significantly between the 1870s and 1890s (see Figure 3.2). Of the few with prior nursing experience in the early days of the scheme, over 40 per cent came from asylums or workhouse infirmaries, while 20 per cent had experience from one of the large London hospitals. After the 1870s, this latter group disappeared almost completely. This is hardly surprising: such hospitals were also developing probationer schemes, so – except in unusual circumstances – it was highly unlikely that they would move from one training scheme to another.

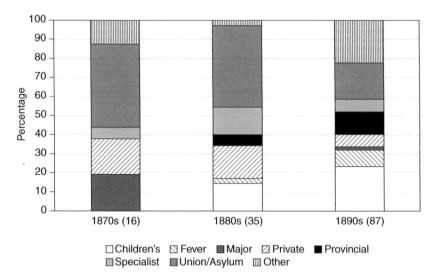

Figure 3.2 Previous nursing experience of probationers at St George's, 1870–1900 (source: St George's Nurses' Database. Children's = children's hospitals; Fever = hospitals under the control of the Metropolitan Asylums Board; Major = major London hospital; Private = working as a private nurse; Provincial = general hospitals outside London; Specialist = hospitals such as the Brompton Hospital for Consumption; Union/Asylum = hospitals associated with workhouses, and asylums for the insane; Other = a range of hospitals including cottage hospitals, army hospitals, hospitals overseas and sisterhoods).

Recruits with workhouse experience also fell off, possibly for similar reasons. Nursing in workhouse infirmaries underwent a slow reform in the second half of the century: trained nurses were being appointed as matrons, and the use of pauper nurses was being phased out. Unions were encouraged by the Poor Law Board to introduce probationer schemes and to develop a career structure for their nurses, and these changes may have rendered it unnecessary for Poor Law nurses to look to the voluntary sector for their training (Ayers 1971; White 1978; Kirby 2002). This explanation needs to be treated with caution: reforms to workhouse nursing proceeded very slowly, and may have been too late to affect recruitment at St George's at this time. However, if workhouse nursing was improving, this could have affected recruitment at St George's from this sector.

The growth in numbers from children's hospitals (and to a lesser extent, provincial institutions) supports Vicinus' claim that women were using such institutions as preliminary training schools (Vicinus 1985). They may even have used these smaller institutions (with their shorter contracts) to experiment with nursing before committing to a longer term at a major hospital, such as St George's.

By the 1890s, probationers with previous nursing experience were the single largest group, but as already mentioned, at the beginning of the scheme domestic service dominated (see Figure 3.3). Housemaids, parlour maids, and general servants were the most common previous positions held (SGHNDB).

These ex-servants formed an attractive prospect – possessing many of the attributes hospital managers were looking for in their new nurse recruits. Familiarity with domestic work would serve them well, as cleaning and scrubbing still formed a significant element of the job. In addition, they would have been habituated to rigid hierarchies, to being the unquestioning recipients of orders, to working extremely long hours and being subject to rigid discipline (Higgs 1986). According to F.M.L. Thompson, the life of a servant was remorseless:

> Their work was ... servile and degrading ... trained to be subordinate, deferential and obsequious, their manners and morals were by definition derivative and imitative, and they lived and worked as isolated individuals in a middle-class world with no opportunities to ... assert their existence as a distinctive subclass.
>
> (Thompson 1988)

Such traits must have been attractive to hospital managers dreaming of a malleable and submissive nursing workforce. Domestic servants would also be very familiar with (and less likely to complain about) the poor-quality accommodation they would find at the hospital, being used to living in

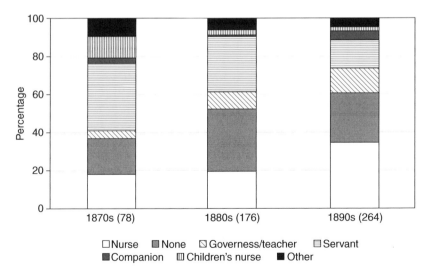

Figure 3.3 Previous occupations of probationers at St George's, 1870–1900 (source: St George's Nurses' Database).

cramped quarters in attics or basements (Perkin 1993). Lacking previous nursing experience, they would have made inefficient assistant nurses, but as probationers they offered a much more attractive proposition to the hospital authorities.

It has been argued that domestic service acted as a bridging occupation, enabling women to move from rural to urban settings where they could acquire experience of middle-class mores and domestic skills (Higgs 1986). The more ambitious could then use such experience to make socially advantageous marriages or to move into other occupations with higher social standing (Higgs 1986). The very public association between nursing and socially elite women, which emerged as the century progressed, must have made it an attractive proposition for domestic servants looking to improve their position in society. The anecdotal evidence, discussed in Chapter 2, that some St George's nurses moved to London to take up domestic service prior to joining the hospital supports this. The fall-off in domestic service recruits in the 1890s is a reflection of the changing social profile of the Nursing Department: as more middle-class women entered the hospital, the proportion with this previous work experience would also be expected to fall. Within working-class recruits, however, domestic servants still represented over 50 per cent of probationers (SGHNDB).

The growth in recruits with no previous occupation also reflects the rise in recruitment of middle-class women. In the 1870s, they represented less than 20 per cent of all probationers, but this figure leapt to over one third in the 1880s. Those who entered with no previous employment in the 1870s tended to be either married or widowed, but a decade later the majority was single, representing 'the better class of candidates' the hospital was attempting to entice. By the 1890s, 80 per cent of probationers with no previous occupation came from the top two social classes (SGHNDB).

In addition to improving the character of the Nursing Department, the new probationer scheme was also expected to address high turnover among assistant nurses, which blighted the Department in the 1850s and 1860s. Assistant nurses brought unacceptable habits from other institutions and did not stay long enough to learn good ones; nursing was inefficient and discipline was poor as a result. The new probationer scheme, by providing a pool of self-trained, prospective assistant nurses (and by default, head nurses), was intended to remedy these problems. It appeared to be successful. The Committee of Nursing stated in 1878 that the new scheme was creating a large staff of:

> Women trained by ourselves to select from for the higher grades, & ... as a general rule those so trained & found worthy of promotion are more likely to give satisfaction than [those] introduced from other institutions.

> (SGHWB/42, 24 April 1878)

In further proof that the scheme was also improving the quality of recruits, the Committee of Nursing reported in 1881:

> We continue to get a better class of candidates than formerly; the nurses have been well conducted and [none of the probationers] has been discharged for inebriety or other grave moral offences.
>
> (SGHWB/45, 13 April 1881)

By 1882, the only nurses dismissed for misconduct had been recruited from other hospitals, suggesting that, indeed, the main problems with discipline and poor behaviour could be overcome by staffing the hospital with its own probationers (SGHWB/47 4 April 1883).

Probationer schemes were used by all major hospitals as a way of improving the quality of nursing, but most took them one step further. At Bart's, St Thomas', King's College, University College, the London, the Middlesex and Guy's, the governors saw opportunities to bolster finances by charging women to train as nurses, through 'paying probationer' schemes (Morten 1892). To attract women to such schemes, they were often offered preferential treatment, both in terms of duties undertaken and accommodation provided. At Guy's, there was a strict division between regular and paying (or lady) probationers. The former received certificates after three years and were eligible only for staff nurse positions, while the 'ladies' trained for one year and immediately became eligible for promotion to ward sister. Lady probationers were housed in separate accommodation and excused night duty (*H/NM*, 19 September 1896).

St George's did not follow this route. As it was in the same (precarious) financial position as other voluntary hospitals of the period, it is surprising that it chose not to tap into this source of additional income. The absence of paying probationers is even harder to understand considering the stream of requests to the hospital from ladies wishing to gain experience in nursing. Ladies were admitted throughout the period to observe or learn nursing, but with no evidence that they paid any fees.[24] Most were admitted on vague terms, but some came with more specific requirements. In 1861, Mrs Lancaster wrote requesting that she and her assistants be allowed to attend 'for the purpose of learning the practical duties of nursing', being about to open a convalescent home in nearby Brompton Square (SGHWB/31, 22 May 1861).[25] Other institutions made similar requests in the 1850s and 1860s, sometimes acceded to and sometimes not. One of the reasons for rejecting applicants was a lack of accommodation. Mrs Edwards wrote from Bath asking permission to 'send in respectable women ... to St George's as pupil nurses to be trained for the space of three or six months [but] not engaged in & wasting their powers in scrubbing' (SGHWB/33, 25 April 1866). She reassured the hospital that her nurses were from respectable middle-class homes, 'sufficiently well educated to meet the requirement of the Medical Staff', but emphatically did not form a sisterhood (SGHWB/33, 25 April 1866). The Board agreed to accept the women, providing they found their own accommodation (SGHWB/33, 25 April 1866). Mrs Edwards was probably right to distance herself from sisterhoods; four years previously a similar request from St Margaret's Convent in East Grinstead had been rejected (SGHWB/32, 22 January 1862).[26]

Institutional applications for training places diminished once the hospital established its own probationer scheme – perhaps the growth in numbers of internal probationers made it more difficult to accommodate trainees from the outside. However, applications from individual women, often supported by influential figures and local residents, continued. In 1872, Lord Ossington (John Evelyn Denison, retired speaker of the House of Commons) petitioned the Weekly Board on behalf of his niece, Miss Denison, who was subsequently admitted 'to learn nursing' (SGHCON/1, 18 November 1872). In the 1840s, he had lived close to the hospital (in Upper Grosvenor Street), which may explain his connection with it (Barker 2004). In 1884, Mademoiselle La Baronne d'Ablaing[27] applied to be admitted to learn nursing (SGHCON/1, 14 July 1884); and, in 1875, Mrs Bouverie asked if her daughter could be admitted to learn nursing for 'a few hours a day' (SGHCON/1, 15 February 1875). She was probably Mrs Edward Pleydell Bouverie, wife of a Whig politician whose family lived in Wilton Crescent, just behind the hospital (Boase 2004).

In addition to local dignitaries, medical men connected to the hospital also used their position to secure admission for female relatives (or potential private employees) to learn nursing. In 1870, Dr Reginald Thompson (who trained at St George's and held the post of Registrar there in the 1860s) wrote that he would 'like to send a Lady, Miss Helen Watson, to the hospital to learn nursing' (SGHWB/35, 19 January 1870; Plarr 1930: 166). She was accepted on the understanding that she would be 'under the direction of the Apothecary and the Matron' (SGHCON/1, 24 January 1870).

There is no evidence to suggest that any of these women who came 'for a few hours a day' paid for the privilege; and it seems unlikely that they intended to make a career of it. More likely, they were curious to experience an occupation which was receiving a great deal of publicity, surrounded, as it was, by an aura of heroism and moral fervour. It could also be argued that a short period of nurse training was viewed as good preparation for young women's future roles as wives and mothers (Rafferty 1996).

In a rare reference to 'special probationers', a petition was laid before the St George's Board in 1873 to allow 'certain Ladies & others desirous of receiving hospital training' to be admitted as trainees (SGHCON/1, 7 April 1873). The original probationer scheme had been in place for four years, and the Committee of Nursing replied that such women could be admitted through the normal channels, but they were required to abide by all the existing rules, including the obligation to sign up for two years

(SGHCON/1, 7 April 1873). It is not obvious why the petitioner felt such 'ladies' merited a special case, and judging by the committee's response, they believed it was not necessary.

Confirmation that ladies could be admitted as full probationers did not stop the flow of women requesting admission on a more informal basis, and they continued to enter for short periods of time, at varying times of the day. By 1883, their numbers must have grown, as the committee decided they needed some regulation – presumably they were interfering with efficiency in the department. Instead of formalizing the arrangements, through a paying probationer scheme, the committee merely limited the number admitted to four at any time, and introduced a requirement to stay for three months (SGHCON/1, 9 April 1883). Whether any women admitted under these conditions went on to join the regular staff of probationers is unknown: the Nurse Registers reveal no evidence to support this. In 1881, a Miss Carey was given permission to enter for three months, with a view to becoming a probationer afterwards, but neither she (nor any of the ladies mentioned above) have entries in the Nurse Registers (SGHCON/1, 11 April 1881), suggesting they never joined the staff.[28]

After the 1883 initiative there were few references to lady nurses in the minutes and no further discussion of lady probationers, until curiously, in 1895, the Committee of Nursing was asked to draw up a set of rules for paying probationers (SGHCON/2, 14 January 1895). There had been no prior discussion of the plan and no action was subsequently taken. The matter was raised again in 1897, and this time a set of rules was published (SGHCON/2, 18 January 1897). The rules were very similar to those for ordinary probationers and contained no special privileges. The fee was set at 13 guineas per quarter. Paying probationers were to live in the same accommodation as the regular nurses, eat the same meals, keep the same hours, and were expected to undertake the same duties as the regular probationers. The main concession was the length of their term: which was to be one year, compared to the obligatory three years for ordinary probationers. Additionally, paying probationers were not obliged to attend lectures or sit exams. One rule – which may give a hint as to the hospital's attitude towards such women – stands out: the requirement to 'conform cheerfully to all the hospital's rules [and] yield implicit obedience to any instruction from the Matron and Sisters' (SGHCON/2, 18 January 1897). This need to 'comply cheerfully' also appears in the rules for special probationers at Bart's ('The Nursing Profession', *NR*, 6 October 1894: 218). It was not included in rules for ordinary probationers at either institution, and suggests that 'specials' might have been prone to sulking or surliness.[29]

Despite the production of these rules, income from fees continued to be absent from hospital accounts, and this is interpreted as the strongest evidence against such a scheme being implemented. Why did St George's not follow its major competitors with regard to paying probationers? In the 1870s and 1880s, most of St George's head nurses were working-class women (as discussed in Chapter 2) and had worked at the hospital for a considerable number of years. The managers may have been concerned that the introduction of a privileged group of probationers would create tensions. Outbreaks of dissent at other hospitals, where lady pupils had been admitted, had been widely publicized, and may have caused St George's governors to be cautious.[30]

They may also have feared the aspirations of lady probationers, having already suffered two negative experiences with such women – Emily Jones (the lady who paid to join the hospital in 1868) and Zepharina Veitch. Both cases (discussed in detail in Chapter 2) had been troublesome and may have given the governors cause for concern when contemplating anything similar on a larger scale. By receiving fees, the hospital would leave itself vulnerable to escalating demands from a group of women likely to be more eloquent and articulate than the regular nurses.

Articles and letters in the nursing press, in the early 1890s, suggest this fear was justified. In 1893, an 'Old-fashioned Matron' wrote of her experience with paying probationers: 'Every day ... was anxiously reviewed by the paying pupils, who were ever on the alert, asking questions, observing much, feeling injured in spirit if after a day on duty they had not acquired fresh knowledge' (*NR*, 25 November 1893: 272). She was in favour of paying probationers, believing them to be more motivated than their non-paying colleagues, but from a manager's point of view, this zeal to learn could be excessive, disruptive and difficult to control.

The arrangement between paying probationers and hospitals was often described as a two-way contract, in which each had legal obligations towards the other (*NR*, 20 November 1890). This was in stark contrast to ordinary probationers, whose contracts were decidedly one-way, to their disadvantage. At St George's, a probationer's employment could be terminated at any time if she disappointed the Committee of Nursing. She, on the other hand, could only break her contract (without penalties applying) with the special permission of the committee (SGHCON/2, 8 May 1899). Paying probationers, on the other hand, had more leverage in their disputes with managers, by dint of the financial relationship which existed between them.

It was also commonly assumed that paying probationers came with hidden costs. According to the *Nursing Record*, women who paid for their training were in a position to make demands: about the quality of training they received, the state of their accommodation, and the chores they were prepared to undertake – or not (*NR*, 17 September 1898). Although ward maids had been introduced into most major hospitals by the end of the century, probationers were still expected to undertake light cleaning duties. An aggrieved probationer wrote to the *Nursing Record* that if probationers were, like medical students, to pay for their training, then presumably, also like medical students, they would not be expected do cleaning (*NR*, 12 March 1898).

Faced with such potential disadvantages, perhaps St George's reluctance to embrace paying probationers can be understood. By the end of the century, even after the appointment of Miss Smedley (who had championed such schemes at the HSC) no further reference to paying probationers had been made. It has been suggested that St George's failed to attract such trainees, losing out to more prestigious training schools, such as St Thomas'. But St George's had an aristocratic reputation – reinforced by its location – which must have made it more attractive (in that respect at least) than other elite London hospitals (K. Waddington, private communication, 2005). The fact that many higher-class women did enrol as ordinary probationers adds further evidence to support the argument that a paying probationer scheme just did not exist. In an institution which prided itself on being run along meritorious lines, there may have been no room for potentially divisive paying probationers.

The structure of nurse training at St George's changed little over the first 20 years. From 1869, when probationers were first admitted, they served a minimum of two years and were paid £12 per annum. They were given uniforms, board and lodging and £2 a year for washing (SGHCON/1, 28 November 1871). Instruction was delivered by head nurses on the wards where they worked. They were expected to serve as assistant nurses when needed and were required to obey all the rules of the hospital (SGHCON/1, 28 November 1871). After one month's trial they signed the following agreement:

> Having now become practically acquainted with the duties required of an Hospital Nurse and having carefully read the rules of the Hospital I hereby agree to comply with the same and to continue in the service of the Hospital for the space of two years from the date of entry, and shall be glad to undertake any situation in the Hospital (before expiration of my term) that the Nursing Committee shall think suitable to my abilities.
>
> (SGHCON/1, 28 November 1871)

This agreement was very important to the hospital. It halted the high turnover among junior nurses and created a guaranteed pool of cheap labour – assistant nurses earned between £18 and £20 a year compared to the £12 earned by their trainee counterparts. In 1872, Probationer Jessica Bendall was ordered to undertake some assistant nurse duties on a temporary basis. She refused to comply, although the order was within the terms of her contract (SGHCON/1, 27 May 1872). Did she feel her position as a trainee was being abused? Her reason for resigning was not recorded, but it is possible.

By 1877, it was deemed necessary to introduce sanctions against women who broke their agreements and a fine of up to one quarter's wages was introduced (SGHCON/1, 14 May 1877). A system of returnable deposits paid by probationers on joining was also introduced: 'Probationers Rosenfield & Carswell are not to be kept on after the first year of training and their deposits will be returned' (SGHCON/1, 9 April 1883). Probationer Whitlock, on the other hand, requested to be released from her contract. Her request was granted 'on condition that she forfeits her deposit' (SGHCON/1, 9 March 1885). Stuart Wildman has reported a similar phenomenon at Birmingham General Hospital, where a forfeitable fee of £21 was introduced for all probationers entering the hospital in 1899 (1999).[31]

In the mid-1870s, in another move that seemed to presage a paying probationer scheme, it was proposed that probationers receive no wages in the first year and only £4 for washing in the second year, with a small wage for those who required it (SGHCON/1, 23 May 1873). Two years later, a two-tier training scheme (reminiscent of schemes at St Thomas' and Guy's) was proposed: probationers to be admitted to train either as assistant or head nurses. The former entered a one-year scheme, while the latter signed up for two (SGHCON/1, 15 February 1875). Taken together, these proposals suggest the hospital was attempting to restrict access to women who could support themselves for at least one year. Although approved by the Weekly Board, the new plans met with strenuous objections from the Medical Committee, and it seems unlikely that they were ever routinely implemented.[32]

In 1885, the length of training increased to three years. In a glowing account of her career, Harriet Coster was credited with being 'one of the first to insist on a three years' standard of training for nurses' (*NR*, 7 April 1894: 228–9). While the three-year scheme was certainly introduced during her tenure, it is unclear what role she played in the decision. Pragmatic reasons of staff retention appeared to have been the driving force, rather than any lofty ideals to improve nurse education. Too many nurses were leaving on completion of their two-year course and receipt of their certificate, and this irritated the Board (SGHWB/49, 22 April 1885). There was no hint that the extension was necessary for enhanced skill acquisition; rather, the managers were annoyed that the hospital was failing to reap the benefits of its investment in nurse training.

Training continued to be of an entirely practical nature. There is no information about the nature of this training, or whether probationers were rotated among the wards, as they were at St Thomas'. However, as great admirers of Nightingale, it is feasible that elements of the St Thomas' system would have been adopted.[33] All that is known about probationers' experience during the 1870s and 1880s is that their day started at 6 a.m., with breakfast at 6.45 a.m. They were on the wards from 7.30 in the morning to 9.30 at night, and were expected to attend daily evening prayers at 10 p.m. (SGHCON/1, 28 November 1871). Training was left entirely in the hands of the head nurses, with no defined curriculum apparent.

Nurse lectures first appeared in 1882, when two of the hospital's surgeons, Clinton Dent and Henry Bennett, offered 'a course of lectures to the nurses upon their duties' (SGHWB/47, 1 November 1882). They were extremely successful, well attended and 'highly appreciated', and marked the beginning of annual nurse lectures, which eventually became an integral part of nurse training (SGHWB/48, 26 March 1884). Attendance was voluntary, but the Committee of Nursing discovered the nurses were keen to participate, 'when they could be spared from duty on the wards' (SGHWB/49, 22 April 1885). In 1889, Dr Dickinson added a short course on 'practical medicine' (SGHWB/52, 10 April 1889). The lecturers gave their time voluntarily; but in 1890, they demanded a fee and the Committee of Nursing, recognizing the growing importance of the lectures, agreed to pay them (SGHCON/2, 6 January 1890). It is questionable as to what value the Weekly Board placed on these lectures in the early days. In 1887, the annual report on nursing extended the committee's thanks to Mr Dent for his lectures which 'continued to be of benefit to the nursing staff', and also to Mr Donkin (another lecturer from the Medical School) for his 'very interesting lecture on Alpine scenery' (SGHWB/50, 6 April 1887). The conflation of these two items in the minutes leaves the impression that the Board considered both to be 'useful entertainment'. The voluntary nature of attendance at the lectures further supports this view.

Whether the initiative for nurse lectures came from the medical staff or from the nurses themselves (given the eagerness with which the lectures were greeted) is not known.[34] Most major London hospitals had introduced nurse lectures by this time, and St George's was in competition with them for nursing staff. The provision of lectures would bolster the hospital's image in the public eye – education and training being very much in vogue generally – and could be used in the ongoing campaign to recruit women of 'a better class'.

In 1889, the hospital opened its nurses' lectures to the general public. The lectures were advertised in *The Lancet* inviting 'persons engaged in nursing' to pay ten shillings to attend the course (SGHCON/1, 4 January 1889). By 1890, they were being advertised more generally and were offered to 'any ladies wishing to attend' and the fee went up to one guinea (SGHCON/2, 12 February 1890). The hospital had finally discovered a revenue stream from its Nursing Department (which was reported in the annual accounts), without any of the disadvantages discussed above. However, the income was very small, ranging from two guineas in 1890 to eight guineas in 1894. The last course of public lectures was held in 1895, by which time attendance for the probationers had become compulsory.

In conjunction with the introduction of lectures, the Weekly Board issued an edict that all probationers should equip themselves, before arriving at the hospital, with a copy of *Domville's Manual for Hospital Nurses*

(SGHCON/1, 22 December 1882; Domville 1888).[35] A slim volume of only 100 pages, it was reviewed in *The Hospital* in 1888 as,

> One of the most concise and thorough works on nursing ever written, and while it will never take the place of fuller teaching, will always be a handy volume to carry about to refresh the memory. ... It is seldom we see a book so devoid of faults, and so much to the point.
>
> (*H/NM*, 21 July 1888: lxiv)

This small book, which was to be required reading for all trainees, was one of a host of nursing textbooks published in the late nineteenth century. Ann Bradshaw's analysis of nineteenth-century nurse training manuals concluded that a typical manual was organized in three main sections. Initial chapters stressed the moral imperative of nursing. This was followed by chapters on anatomy, physiology and diseases and their care, before the main body of the book which concentrated on practical nursing (Bradshaw 2000).

Domville's Manual does not conform to Bradshaw's analysis.[36] Its introductory chapter (a mere four pages in length) says little on vocation or obedience. In the section headed 'The Nurse's Duties as Regards Herself', Domville concentrated on practicalities: the need for a nurse to be neat and tidy in her dress, and quiet in manner. Towards her superiors, the word 'obedience' was not used and, instead, Domville focused on the assistance she could give to medical colleagues. Whilst he warned against undue familiarity between a nurse and her superiors, he did not proscribe her from discussing a doctor's course of treatment, merely reminding her not to do so in front of the patient (Domville 1888).

Without knowing how widely used these different manuals were, it is difficult to assess the significance of their content. Two copies of Florence Nightingale's *Notes on Nursing* (laden with references to the moral character of nursing) were available to St George's nurses in their library, but it was the more practical book which they were required to have with them at all times. Bradshaw's analysis of nursing textbooks supports the notion that nursing was a vocation, but it must be asked if the main purpose of these manuals was to promote this view, rather than to be used as practical instruction guides for nurses on the wards. Evidence from St George's demonstrates that, given the choice, managers opted for the practical over the theoretical.

Domville's lack of reference to vocation or Christian motive for nurses' work chimes with the hospital's apparent non-denominational character. Its relationship with various sisterhoods, already discussed, supports this; and the *Nursing Record's* advice to Roman Catholic women – that St George's was one of only a small group of London hospitals which would accept them to train as nurses – provided further evidence of its non-denominational stance (*NR*, 1 August 1889).[37] In addition, the hospital's rule which required nurses to attend the hospital's chapel, or 'other suitable place if not Church of England', indicated a willingness to accept non-Anglicans (SGHCON/2, 10 March 1898).

Another differentiating feature of *Domville's* is a lack of theoretical content. Unlike most of the books studied by Bradshaw, it is completely devoid of any discussion of human anatomy or physiology; neither are there chapters on diseases and their care. Instead, it focuses entirely on the practicalities of carrying out a variety of nursing procedures, such as how to undress an accident patient (two and half pages) and instructions on leeching and cupping. The level of detail indicates that the book was intended for practical instruction. An example on 'wet-sheet packing' demonstrates this,

> Cover the bed with a sheet of waterproofing; on it lay three or more large blankets (not doubled); on these place the patient, lying on his side; then dip a sheet in the water of the required temperature, wring it, fold three or four times, and apply along the back; turn the patient over, then apply a sheet similarly prepared over the front of the body; then turn over the blankets previously left overlapping, and wrap the patient in the them, adding a coverlet or additional blanket. The patient should remain in the pack for 20, 30, 45 or 60 minutes, as ordered.
>
> (Domville 1888: 35)

The reader is given no theory behind the procedure, no explanation of the conditions in which it is used, nor the likely outcome of such treatment. It simply instructs the nurse, in a step-by-step manner, how to perform the task. Does this indicate a reluctance on the part of the hospital to encourage theoretical learning in its nurses? The late introduction of lectures (and their voluntary nature for over ten years) seems to support that interpretation. On the other hand, this type of practice (the blind following of instruction) is contrary to *The Manual's* earlier encouragement of nurses to ask questions of the doctor. Perhaps, as a doctor himself, Domville was only too aware of his colleagues' desire to control nurses' access to theoretical knowledge. His book left this firmly in the hands of the medical staff of hospitals; it was the duty of doctors to instil the appropriate level of theory in their nurses, while the book served as an *aide memoire* to its practical application.

A clear example of censorship of nurses' knowledge by doctors is found in a manual originally written for American nurses. In the English version, Dyce Duckworth wrote:

> In preparing [this book] for use amongst British nurses, it has been necessary to alter the text in certain parts. ... Some of the instruction ... appeared to be designed with the object of training an irregular

order of medical and surgical practitioners ... calculated to encourage nurses to prescribe for patients ... and [assume] other serious responsibilities. Such instruction has been rigidly excluded.

(Duckworth 1897: vii–viii)

By using *Domville's Manual*, devoid of theoretical content, the dangers of accidently exposing nurses to too much medical knowledge could be avoided.

If the choice of instruction manual is representative of the hospital's approach to nurse education in the early 1880s, then one can conclude that its nurses were required to be highly skilled in a variety of procedures, neat and tidy in their dress and method of working, observant and questioning of their role, but not schooled in theory of disease or its treatment.

Attendance at lectures continued to be voluntary into the 1890s. By 1891, the lectures had been expanded to include elementary anatomy, physiology, surgical and medical nursing, air and ventilation, infection and disinfection and children's nursing (SGHWB/53, 1 April 1891). Practical instruction remained in the domain of head nurses, who decided individually what and when a probationer should be taught. A patient's complaint that his nurse did not know how to take a temperature properly was a clear manifestation of this arbitrary approach to training. The Weekly Board responded immediately by ordering all new probationers, on entering the hospital, to receive instruction on temperature taking from a medical officer (SGHWB/53, 18 June 1890).

Up to this point, there had been no formal examinations, but in 1894, nurse exams were finally introduced. They had been a feature in most major London hospitals since the late 1880s, and it is difficult to interpret the delay at St George's, except as yet further evidence of the managers' reluctance to embrace nurse education. The introduction of exams coincided with the gathering pace of the registration debate, and this seems to be no coincidence. London teaching hospitals generally opposed a central system of nurse registration, and had announced their opposition to it in 1888 (*H/NM*, 14 April 1888: 26). They were reluctant to hand influence over nurse training to a central body, and were determined to maintain control over every aspect of their nursing departments, including who should be recruited, what they should be taught and what standards were required for qualification. The hospitals argued that their systems were the only guarantee of high standards, and that a central system (which would by definition bring in other less prestigious institutions) would necessarily lead to a decline (Witz 1992: Rafferty 1996). St George's was among this elite group, but in 1888 had neither compulsory lectures nor examinations. It had to review its nurse training programmes to avoid providing ammunition for the pro-registration lobby.

The new exams tested candidates on what they had learned on the wards and from the lectures 'they may have attended during their 12 months training' (SGHCON/2, 19 February 1894). The length of training stated here contradicted previous statements, but reveals a common practice in London hospitals. Women signed two- or three-year probationer contracts but were moved to junior nurse positions after only a year. This practice was at the heart of the London Hospital controversy in the early 1890s, when it was accused of sending out only half-trained probationers (that is, those with one year's training) to fulfil lucrative private contracts. Eva Luckes argued that her nurses were fully trained after one year, but required the second year to gain further practical experience (HoLSC/MH 1890). It is clear that St George's managers took a similar view.

The introduction of nurse exams immediately exposed the flawed nature of St George's training scheme, in particular the unsystematic approach to practical skills acquisition. Nurses sat a written examination of eight questions and a *viva voce*. They were tested on anatomy and physiology, practical aspects of medical and surgical nursing and their practical skills in bandaging. The first examiners' reports were devastating, but they excused the disappointing performance on the lack of experience in exam technique. Sitting exams was a novel experience for many of the women, who 'were afflicted with a not unnatural nervousness, which in some cases rendered them almost incapable of doing themselves justice' (SGHCON/2, 11 June 1894).

The poor performance in practical nursing was blamed on a lack of organized instruction. Examiners noted that both nurses and their teachers were being tested, and concluded that 'the systematic instruction by senior nurses ... is very far from being as complete as it should be' (SGHCON/2, 11 June 1894). On bandaging, one of the most deficient areas, they said 'the probationers ought at the outset of their career to have demonstrations ... and not be allowed to pick up their knowledge as best they can' (SGHCON/2, 11 June 1894).

As late as 1894, systematic training of probationers was still non-existent. There were no lists of tasks in which probationers had to demonstrate efficiency, as Nightingale had introduced at St Thomas', nor any system of checking that they had received instruction in basic nursing procedures (Woodham-Smith 1950). Instead, the practical training of probationers continued entirely at the whim of the head nurse. The examining doctors concluded there was an urgent need for systematic nurse instruction, for 'it is impossible for them to attain any real proficiency unless they are shown at the outset how to set about their work in the right way' (SGHCON/2, 2 June 1894).

Mrs Coster, while being sympathetic towards the findings, appeared incapable of addressing them. She agreed, after the first set of exams, that she 'had long felt that some systematic teaching of the probationers was necessary, but the work in [my] department has of late years so greatly increased that it has been impossible for [me] to give this' (SGHCON/2, 18 June 1894).

While Coster may have been overburdened, particularly with house-keeping work, it was also true that she was over 60 years old and had been in post for 22 years. Even if she was sympathetic to the enormous changes needed, she may have been too weary to implement them. She may also have been too set in her ways, which had developed in a very different era. Her appointment as Nurse Honorary Secretary to the RBNA, after her retirement from St George's, also suggests a lack of sympathy with the reformers' objectives. By this time, the RBNA was actively campaigning against nurse registration – and in taking on her new role, Coster demonstrated that her sympathies probably did not lie with pro-educationalists.

In the wake of this first experience, the lecture courses became compulsory for the first time. Rules on promotion also changed: probationers now had to serve for at least two years and pass their exams before being promoted to staff nurse (SGHCON/2, 7 May 1894). And, although eligible for promotion after two years, they did not receive the all important certificate until they had successfully completed three years' service. Three classes of certificate were awarded – class 1 (very satisfactory), class 2 (satisfactory) or class 3 (certificate of proof of training and general good conduct) – depending on performance in the exam and a report from the Superintendent of Nursing on the probationer's conduct and efficiency (SGHCON/2, 18 June 1894). This last was a nod in the direction of those concerned that the moral basis of nursing was being eroded by a focus on acquisition of theoretical knowledge.

By 1896, the doctors reported that the lectures and exams were having a beneficial effect. They gave probationers an incentive to work and encouraged them to make better use of the learning opportunities presented by a large teaching hospital (SGHCON/2, 9 March 1896). But bandaging and splint-making remained a thorn in the side. After one set of exams, the examiners again blamed the teachers for nurses' poor performance in bandaging, a comment which was repeated in 1898 (SGHCON/2, 9 March 1896, 14 August 1898). Quite why it proved so problematic was not discussed, but a lack of a coordinated syllabus of instruction suggests such elements could easily be overlooked.

Probationers had to wait for the appointment of Miss Smedley, in 1897, before a systematic scheme was introduced. She brought a wealth of experience in the 'new style of nursing' – gained during her training at Bart's and her experience at the HSC – and was quite a contrast to the old Matron. The speed with which her reforms were implemented suggests that the Nursing Department had fallen into a moribund state. Having once been at the forefront of nursing reform, St George's had lost its momentum. An article on nursing at the hospital in 1897 described Mrs Coster as belonging to 'the older school of Matrons' and compared the nursing system at St George's with the 'more modern' hospitals such as St Thomas', King's or the London (*H/NM*, 7 August 1897: 168).

Smedley was a shining light of reform. Her new probationer scheme bore many resemblances to the one she had introduced at the HSC during her reign as Lady Superintendent. For the first time, the three-year probationary period had a defined structure and timetable. It included lessons from the sisters in practical nursing, given on the wards and in class demonstrations, on subjects such as washing patients, making beds, giving enemata and baths, and simple bandaging. These subjects formed the basis of the first year. In the second and third years, probationers attended theory classes from the medical staff and demonstrations of more complex nursing procedures by the sisters. A practical exam during the first year was followed by theory and practical exams in the third year. Progess through each stage depended on passing exams; passing the third-year exam resulted in the probationer being promoted to staff nurse, and the award of the certificate (SGHCON/2, 3 March 1898).

In 1898, the probation department underwent a further important reform, with the restriction of entry to certain times of the year. Prior to this, new probationers joined as they presented themselves. By limiting the new intake to once every three months, the hospital created groups of women who were all at the same level in their nurse education, following the same course of instruction (SGHCON/2, 10 March 1898).

In a final major alteration, which completed the overhaul of nurse training, overall responsibility for probationers was placed firmly in the hands of the matron. Although the sisters still supervised and taught probationers on their wards, the matron was responsible for the quality and organization of their training. To strengthen this further, probationer accommodation – which since the early 1890s had been located at some distance from the main site – was moved back to Hyde Park Corner, bringing probationers under the matron's direct and constant supervision (SGHCON/2, 14 February 1898, 21 March 1898).

Thus, by the end of the nineteenth century, St George's could finally be said to have an established nurse training school, along the lines of other London teaching hospitals. The hospital was at least ten years behind its competitors in attaining this milestone, and much of the responsibility for this long delay would appear to lie at Mrs Coster's door. Her lack of sympathy with a more enlightened form of nurse education (suggested by her position in the RBNA) illuminates her period of tenure as Superintendent of Nurses at St George's. Ethel Fenwick interpreted her support for the RBNA as evidence of a willingness to submit to medical authority; and it could be that such an attitude was exactly what appealed to St George's governors when they appointed her, given their unsettling experience with Miss Veitch.

Conclusion

It is no coincidence that nurse education developed at a time of increasing focus on the training of young women for occupations through which they could support themselves. It has also been linked to an emerging interest in education on the part of young women and identified as an element in the drive to gentrify nursing and as a response to the increasingly scientific nature of medicine. But there may have been a more prosaic rationale for its rise to prominence in the mid- to late nineteenth century. For hospital managers, facing growing patient numbers, an insatiable demand for beds and increasingly stretched finances, the introduction of nurse training, paradoxically, offered a way to alleviate some of those pressures.

The development of probationer training at St George's was more a process of evolution than revolution. The initial impetus came from the need for a large pool of internally trained nurses, to address issues of discipline and nurse turnover. In the early days, applicants from a domestic service background were favoured, considered to be more malleable than women who had worked in other large institutions, where they might have acquired bad habits. Later, the preference shifted away from the servant class towards women with a more middle-class background and a better education, more able to cope with new developments in theoretical training.

At hospitals, such as St Thomas', there was a heavy emphasis on moral training of nurses and the vocational nature of the work was stressed, but this does not seem to be the case at St George's. The use of *Domville's Manual*, a very practical instruction guide devoid of spiritual or religious overtones, supports this. Although probationers were required to attend evening prayers and chapel on Sundays, this requirement was quickly diluted by the needs of the hospital, to the point that, in 1894, the obligation was completely removed.[38]

Until the arrival of Miss Smedley, and with the exception of Miss Veitch, the matrons at St George's had a small voice in the development of the Nursing Department. Arrangements were the preserve of the Committee of Nursing (composed of hospital governors and a small number of medical officers) which grew in power and influence over the latter decades of the nineteenth century. Its Chairman for most of this period was Hugh Macpherson, a retired army surgeon, who had trained at St George's, and who took a close interest in nursing at the hospital. The Matron's involvement in the committee was marginal. She was not a voting member, but was called to give evidence when needed. Her involvement was restricted to attempts to influence decisions, rather than to make them. Lindsay Granshaw has argued that the contribution of medical men to the development of nursing has been of less importance than that of laymen and women. She cites St Thomas', where the Treasurer was very influential in the decision to accommodate Nightingale's training school within his hospital, as an example of this (Granshaw 1981). Similarly, Sir Sidney Waterlow (Treasurer at Bart's) and Sydney Holland (Chairman of the Hospital Committee at the London) played key roles in persuading their hospitals to develop systematic training for their nurses (Collins and Parker 2003; Yeo 1995). At St George's, though, medical members of the Committee of Nursing took an active role in its business, and evidence suggests that the original impetus for nurse education came from them (Helmstadter 2002).[39]

At St George's, training focused (if that is the right description) on the acquisition of practical nursing skills and paid scant attention to theoretical learning until late in the nineteenth century. Even practical training was very hit and miss, left to the whim of ward sisters. The persistence of this 'old-fashioned' approach may be, in part, due to the presence of Mrs Coster. Other hospitals, where theoretical nurse education was introduced earlier, had young, ambitious matrons with 'modern' ideas about nurse education. At such hospitals formal lectures and examinations were well established before St George's began its experiment.

There has been little written about the content of nurse training, or how theory and practical were balanced. However, it seems likely that even where hospitals boasted of the theoretical content of their nurse training, the majority of learning took place on the wards – either at the side of experienced nurses, or occasionally by observing visiting doctors. Although doctors disagreed on the level of medical education a nurse should have, most supported its inclusion, to some extent, in the nursing curriculum. They could appreciate the benefits a nurse with a grounding in medical science could contribute to their own practice, as long as it was carefully controlled.

Certificates of training, awarded on successful completion of courses and examinations, became increasingly important as the century progressed. As one commentator noted, a certificate 'is as important to a nurse as a doctor's is to him', while another compared the value of a nurse's certificate to that of a degree for a clergyman (*NR*, 22 September 1892: 773; 7 July 1894: 12). A hierarchy of certificates developed, which placed the London teaching hospitals at the pinnacle, leaving nurses who trained at provincial establishments disadvantaged in the search for employment. Nurses without certificates were in the worst position, and one wrote to *The Hospital*, urging the Hospital Association to hold exams for such nurses so they too could obtain a certificate (*H/NM*, 21 January 1888; Maggs 1983).

The training schemes, and their resulting highly prized certificates, became a passport to a career that offered, at the very least, the means of independent support. The adventurous used their training to travel abroad, taking their new found skills to far-flung outposts of the Empire. The ambitious used it to construct a career path which incorporated increasing levels of responsibility culminating, for a few, in the highest posts. The next two chapters will investigate how women were able to make use of these newly acquired skills, build careers and ultimately create independent lives for themselves, in a society which, in theory, offered nothing but opprobrium, scorn or pity to the single woman.

Pen Portrait 3 Ann Moseley – nursing as a route to respectability

Ann Moseley, born in Derbyshire in 1844, was the daughter of a higgler (a Victorian door-to-door salesman). She left home in her teens to work as a servant in Birmingham, but by 1866, she was back and with a son – but unmarried. Like so many women in her situation, Ann had to find care for her son, and work to support them both. Her married sister stepped into the breach, while Ann set about earning a living. In 1872 she found work at Lower Clapton Asylum, in London, as housemaid to the Matron, and three years later she joined St George's as an assistant nurse. She probably hid her child from the hospital: the managers were prepared to hire widows with young children but the same latitude would not have been shown to a single mother.

Ann was a good learner, and after only three years was promoted to head nurse. She ran three wards containing 36 patients, two assistant nurses and one probationer. This was a real achievement. Vacancies for head nurse arose infrequently, and competition must have been fierce. She was well regarded by her colleagues. One of the hospital's medical officers said of her:

> 'I had under my care ... in Queen's Ward a young woman ... suffering severely from inflammation of the lungs: in fact ... I despaired of her life ... I remarked to Nurse Moseley that the only chance of saving [her] was by careful nursing. The patient hung between life & death for three days when symptoms of improvement became manifest. ... Now I happen to know that after my remark ... that Nurse Moseley never left her patient, that she gave up to her the time allowed to nurses for recreation & that she did not go down to dinner during the three days on which my patient was so ill.
>
> (SGHNR/2 Moseley)

Praise indeed for a dedicated nurse. Ann left St George's in 1883, 'at her own desire'. She next surfaced in the 1891 census, described as a 'medical nurse'. She was probably working as private nurse. Private nursing freed Ann to live with her family again: in 1891 she was back in Derbyshire living with her son who was now married, with a young daughter. In 1901, the family was still together: Ann, now 57, had given up nursing and was running her own confectionery/bakery shop, probably funded by her savings. For the first time, she was described as a widow. Whether this was a mistake, a piece of etiquette, or an attempt to cover up her dubious past cannot be known.

Ann was able to use nursing to rise up from humble beginnings, but more importantly was able to overcome the stigma of illegitimacy. Her story illustrates the importance of family support when crises struck; and her final choice of occupation illustrates the path retired nurses often took, using their savings to set up a gentle business which could support them in retirement.

4 'Treat your good nurses well'

During the second half of the nineteenth century there was a new public concern for conditions endured by a large percentage of workers. In the late 1880s and early 1890s, this extended to nurses. An article in the *Pall Mall Gazette* – 'White Slavery in Hospitals' – triggered a nationwide public debate on the state of nursing. According to the *Gazette*, a nurse's day was excessively long, dominated by repetitive, physically draining chores, few breaks and no time for meals: 'from seven in the morning until nine at night. Hurry scurry – no rest, no relaxation, almost always on their feet' (*Pall Mall Gazette*, 3 April 1889: 3). Of their living conditions, the article was no more generous: 'A meagre meal … [then] off to bed in a large dormitory with the barest accommodation, and in winter so cold they cast their cloaks and day clothes upon the bed for the purposes of warmth' (*Pall Mall Gazette*, 3 April 1889: 3).

The article whipped a storm of correspondence (not confined to the *Gazette*) from nurses, doctors and patients, affirming its accuracy from personal experience. But equal numbers claimed the opposite, and the *Nursing Record*, in particular, took great exception to the sentiments expressed. Its editorials and letters left no doubt where it stood on the issue:

> I … thank you for the very spirited way in which the Editorial columns of … Nursing Record have taken up the subject of 'White Slavery' … There has been far too much of 'sham sentiment' … about Nurses and their profession. … Our hours are long, and the work is exceedingly arduous. … But taking everything into account – hard work, ill health, and all other 'grievances' of a Nurses life – I think there are very few who would, or do, give it up unless absolutely obliged.
>
> (*NR*, 25 April 1889: 271)

How did nursing become associated with such an emotive term as 'white slavery', with the exploitative and degrading images it conjures up? The origins of the phrase are traced to earlier in the century, when public concern for the welfare of workers was reflected in a raft of Acts of

Parliament directed at improving their lot.[1] Initially, the focus was on children and women working in factories, mines and workshops, but it was gradually extended so that: 'All workers of both sexes began to benefit from Parliament's cautious willingness to enforce minimum standards of health and safety' (Best 1979 [1985]: 137). Improvements were not universally implemented and large swathes of the working population – in small industries, shops, laundries and domestic service – were without any official protection from exploitation (Best 1979 [1985]).

From the 1850s, articles appeared in the press describing the plight of groups of workers toiling in appalling conditions for paltry wages. An example from *The Times* (in 1853) illustrates the mood:

> The facts which led to the Ten Hours Factory Bill had impressed themselves on the public mind to an extent that had hardly been paralleled. Yet, while everyone was rejoicing over the success of that measure, white slavery still existed amongst us.
>
> (*The Times*, 2 March 1853: 8)[2]

This was the first use of the phrase 'white slavery' in *The Times*, in the context of working practices. It was deliberately chosen. The Abolition of Slavery Act had only been passed some 20 years earlier, and in the USA slavery was still legal. Furthermore, it was also associated, in the public's prurient imagination, with a rumoured trade in young European women to Ottoman harems. It was therefore especially shocking when used to describe conditions endured by female workers. Over the following 50 years, the phrase was employed to great oratorical effect to describe conditions in occupations as diverse as locksmiths, omnibus employees, match girls and bar workers. It was invoked frequently in the press to describe the plight of shop assistants, forced to work extremely long hours, constantly on their feet, with few breaks and little reward (*The Times*, 17 April 1882; *The Times*, 9 October 1885: 14; Besant 1888).

'White slavery' became synonymous with another equally evocative term, 'sweating'.[3] 'Sweating' referred to a group of industries notorious for very low wages, long hours and insanitary working conditions; populated by unskilled or semi-skilled labourers often working from their own meagre homes (Morris 1986). It was particularly associated with the mass-market clothing business, where home-workers were employed (usually on a piecework basis) to perform single unskilled tasks, such as hemming shirts. It was also used to describe many other piecework occupations: mass-production of furniture, chains and nails all came into this category (G.S. Jones 1971: 107).

Wages were appallingly low. Home-workers in the mass-tailoring trade could earn as little as five shillings a week. The average for women in the London ready-made industry was seven shillings and nine pence (Morris 1986).[4] With social commentators defining a subsistence wage as 25 shillings a week for men and 14 to 16 shillings for women, female workers in the mass-clothing industry were clearly being paid poverty rates (quoted in Morris 1986).[5]

In 1888, the public outcry against such exploitation resulted in a House of Lords Select Committee to investigate the 'Sweating System'. The committee's deliberations culminated in a series of reports published in 1889 and 1890, which provided evidence of sweating in many occupations (HoLSC/SS 1888–90).

The committee's report raised awareness of working conditions in a range of industries, not just those selected for investigation, and in this atmosphere, perhaps it is not surprising that nurses should join the debate. Their hours were notoriously long and their wages low, and they were quick to capitalize on the public mood for reform. There was never any serious question that nursing was a 'sweated industry', but nevertheless, many wrote to the newspapers complaining of their own conditions, evoking the 'sweating' debate in their defence. They saw reflections of themselves in the sweated industries and appeared to set out quite purposefully to use the debate to bring their own issues to the public's attention. In reality, nurses' working conditions bore little resemblance to the sweated trades, and in terms of low pay – which the House of Lords Committee gave particular weight to in defining 'sweating' – there was no comparison (Morris 1986).

A probationer earned £10 to £12 a year, the equivalent of three shillings and three pence to four shillings and seven pence a week; which would seem to place them firmly within the definition of a 'sweated trade'. But any comparisons must also include the value of board and lodging, provided by hospitals and estimated to be worth an additional 15 to 19 shillings a week.[6] Added together, this gave even a probationer a total weekly income as high as 24 shillings. Compared to Cadbury and Shann's minimum subsistence wage for women, nurses were relatively well remunerated. Staff nurses, who earned between £20 and £30 a year (plus board and lodging) were on a par with the minimum wage recommended for male workers. Clearly, while nurses' wages were not overly generous, their lot was far removed from that of women working in the sweated industries.[7]

There was more similarity in the number of hours worked, and the conditions of their work and living spaces. Nurses hours stretched from 12 to 14 a day, seven days a week, while home-workers in London's tailoring trade averaged between ten and 16 hours a day; and, while nurses' accommodation and food was provided, the standard of provision was heavily criticized (Morris 1986). There was a clearer correlation between the two groups in this respect, and nurses emphasized hours of work, lack of rest and poor living conditions to strengthen their claim to be participants in the sweating debate.

The campaign to generate public sympathy for nurses' plight was successful, and the 'sweating' of nurses received a great deal of press attention. Interest was stirred by letters from nurses who used the debate to air personal grievances; and the press took up their cause, quick to generate sensationalist headlines, linking the 'sweating' of nurses to the even more emotive 'white slavery'. This was a shocking juxtaposition of degradation and innocence, conflating connotations of sexual exploitation with the purity and innocence more normally associated with nurses.

While the *Nursing Record* took great exception to outsiders – such as the *Pall Mall Gazette* – criticizing the profession, it was not averse to using these emotive terms itself. In a vitriolic attack on Guy's Hospital, in 1892, these same terms were used to stir up public outrage. 'Charitable Sweating' was the headline attached to its editorial, describing how that 'splendid institution' had been turned into 'a commercial concern, grinding the face of its women workers – greedily grasping all it could *sweat* out of its *white slaves*' (*NR*, 3 November 1892: 890, my emphasis).

These debates about nursing came to a head during another Select Committee, this one on metropolitan hospitals, which sat in 1889. The committee's report concluded, among other things, that the case for sweating of nurses had been exaggerated (HoLSC/MH3 1892). The conclusion ignored evidence presented to the committee by several working nurses from the London Hospital, who testified in detail to the extreme hardship and poor treatment suffered by ward nurses there. Rather, it privileged evidence from hospital managers and the Matron (Eva Luckes) who testified to the contrary. It is hardly surprising that the committee favoured the managers' version of events (they were their peers), particularly after accusations by Henry Burdett that pro-registrationists had persuaded those nurses to perjure themselves (*H/NM*, July 1892: 234–6). Neither the managers nor Luckes had anything to gain from acknowledging the nurses' grievances: addressing issues of overwork would inevitably lead to increased costs, and for Luckes (who came in for particular criticism) it was a question of professional pride. Perhaps the nurses' ploy to raise the spectre of the 'sweated' industries had backfired on them; the evidence which emerged from both committees merely served to illustrate how relatively well-off nurses were.

While the sensationalist press reporting of nurses' working conditions reached fever pitch in the early 1890s, individual hospitals had been grappling with the issues for many years. At St George's, poor accommodation, low wages and lack of career prospects had long been identified as obstacles to an efficient nursing department. Throughout the second half of the nineteenth century, the managers sought to stem high turnover among its nursing staff, and its consequent effect on the quality of nursing. The situation was bad: before the 1880s, junior nurses stayed barely long enough to make a meaningful contribution, and the lack of experienced staff generated a increasing use of 'specials', with their associated costs.[8] The increasing complexity of nursing, as medical science advanced, added to this pressure. In consequence, the Management Board was obliged to consider a variety of strategies to introduce more stability into the Nursing Department. Some were coercive, such as the introduction of probationer contracts (already discussed in Chapter 3), which bound them to the hospital for increasing lengths of time. Other strategies were more subtle, designed to encourage trained nurses to remain for longer periods. A policy of internal recruitment (which promised a career structure and promotion), a series of reforms to improve the living conditions, and monetary incentives for long service all fall within this category.

This chapter will discuss whether improvements in nurses' working conditions were driven more by market forces and the hospital's need to be competitive in the recruitment marketplace, than by any altruistic motives regarding nurses' well-being. It will also show nurses in a new light, exercising agency in the initiation of these improvements, rather than being merely passive recipients.

The revolving door

During the 1870s, St George's lost, on average, one third of its regular nurses every year, with over 40 per cent staying for less than 12 months.[9] The size of the problem is illustrated in Figure 4.1.

The annual attrition rates for regular nurses reached a peak between 1875 and 1880, when on average 35 per cent left every year. The figure hides an even starker picture in certain years: in 1872 and 1878 nearly 50 per cent left for one reason or another. Such high turnover left wards in

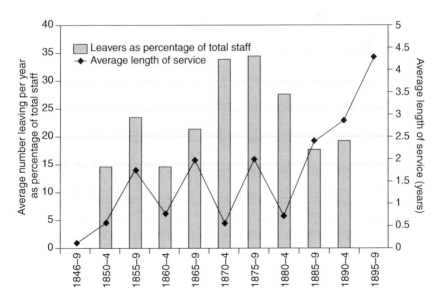

Figure 4.1 Analysis of turnover and length of service of nurses at St George's, 1846–99 (sources: St George's Hospital Nurses' Database).

the care of women with little nursing experience, supervised by increasingly overstretched head nurses. The stress placed on head nurses by this constant flow of semi-trained women must have been vexing. The rapid turnover in staff must also have caused recruitment problems. The supply of promising nurse candidates was not bottomless, and the hospital was often obliged to employ women who – in other circumstances – would have been rejected. Those recruited out of desperation, rather than suitability, were unlikely to stay for any length of time, adding to the crisis. The revolving door's momentum was maintained by this seemingly unbreakable cycle.

The changing nature of service at the hospital is starkly illustrated in Figure 4.2. For the first 40 years of this study the majority of regular nurses left after only one year's service, while only 10–15 per cent stayed for more than three. This pattern was completely reversed by the 1890s, when three to five years' service became the norm. What was behind this emphatic shift?

The increased length of service coincided with the introduction of three-year contracts for probationers, in 1886. Two-year contracts, introduced for the first probationers, had little effect on overall stability in the Nursing Department. Probationer numbers were so small in the 1860s and 1870s that enforced two-year terms had little impact on departmental average length of service. Regular nurses – who made up the majority – were never subject to the same contractual constraints, and were free to leave when they chose, which they continued to do. But as the numbers of probationers rose, the effect of fixed-term contracts became more dramatic and introduced a new stability into the Nursing Department.[10]

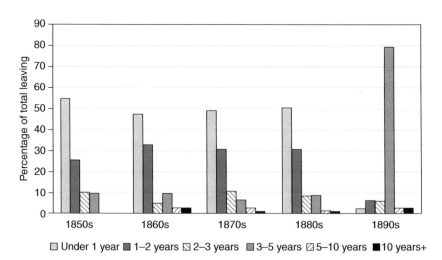

Figure 4.2 Length of service of regular nurses at St George's, by decade (sources: St George's Hospital Nurses' Database, 1840–1900).

When combined with a policy of internal recruitment of probationers to vacant ward nurse positions, the result was an inevitable increase in the average length of service in the Nursing Department as a whole.

Problems of turnover among head nurses were never so acute. Average length of service for this group ranged from four to 11 years: at least 14 head nurses served for over ten years, while five had served for over 20. The introduction of new contracts had no impact on their length of service either. Like regular nurses, they had open contracts, obliged only to work a period of notice before leaving.[11]

On the surface, the head nurses seemed content but further analysis of the data reveals there were some serious problems among this group too. The data in Table 4.1 compares the average length of service to the median for each decade of study, and reveals a crisis in the 1870s.

Although the average length of service for head nurses in the 1870s was four years, the median value indicates that half of those who left had worked at the hospital for less than two. This level of turnover among nurse managers – which was unprecedented – was most acute between 1870 and 1872; instead of losing, on average, three or four head nurses a year, eight left in 1872 alone, five in the same month. This mass exodus coincided with arrival of a new Superintendent of Nurses.

In attempting to understand the events of 1871–2 it is necessary to delve into the circumstances surrounding Maria Gregory's appointment and reign. Gregory joined the hospital in 1869 as a head nurse, and was appointed – in a temporary capacity – as Superintendent of Nursing after only a few months. The appointment was controversial. She was a compromise choice after the committee failed to elect the 'preferred candidate'; and she was too young to be appointed officially, being some months short of the minimum age of 30.[12] Her close association with Zepharina Veitch (her predecessor) was probably her final Achilles' heel – as far as existing staff were concerned. Recruited during Veitch's short but tempestuous reign, it is likely that to the old head nurses she represented a continuation of that regime.

Table 4.1 Statistical analysis of length of service of head nurses at St George's, 1850s–90s

Decade left	Average length of service (years)	Median length of service (years)	No. of head nurses leaving per decade	Average no. of head nurses on staff
1850s	4.1	3.3	14	16
1860s	11.3	8.1	13	19
1870s	4.1	1.9	34	15
1880s	7.4	5.5	23	15
1890s	6.7	5.9	16	21

Source: St George's Hospital Nurses' Database, 1840–1900.

Gregory's lack of experience, her young age and the knowledge that she had been a compromise candidate, probably created tensions between her and her head nurses. Evidence indicates that she struggled to exert authority over them. Her handling of a minor dispute over their breakfast arrangements illustrates this.

To improve discipline in the Nursing Department, the Weekly Board broke with custom, instructing head nurses to take breakfast in the Nurses' Dining Room, rather than in their own rooms (SGHCON/1 18 July 1870). They rebelled against this perceived intrusion into private time, and some refused to comply. After failing to enforce the ruling, Gregory was reduced to falling back on the authority of the Board, producing a written order that further breaches would be reported to the managers (SGHCON/1 29 July 1870). The head nurses were probably testing the authority of their new superintendent; the incident suggests that, after more than six months in post, she had yet to establish control over them.

A further cause of tension originated in plans to open a new wing in 1870, which would add three wards and 36 beds to the hospital (SGHCON/1, 4 July 1870). Gregory was charged by the managers with devising a nursing scheme to accommodate the new wards, without an excessive increase in costs. Her solution was radical. She proposed to reduce the number of head nurses from 18 to 12 (by merging several wards together) and to employ 14 probationers to provide the remaining head nurses with additional support. The plan reduced nursing costs by £50 a year, despite the increase in beds. The additional burden placed on assistant nurses (whose numbers remained static) would be relieved by a team of scrubbers, to take over some of their domestic chores. Even including the cost of scrubbers, Gregory was offering an increase in beds for almost unchanged costs (SGHCON/1, 4 July 1870; SGHWB/35, 6 July 1870).

Tempting as it must have been, the plans were not implemented in full. The three new wards were simply handed to existing head nurses. The increased probationer numbers also failed to materialize – although the team of house servants was strengthened, relieving assistant nurses of some of their more onerous domestic chores (SGHWB/35 6 July 1870). The new regime placed more stress on everyone, but probably hit head nurses hardest, and the mass exodus which took place over the following two years probably reflected dissatisfaction with both the plan and their new leader, who had failed to support and protect their interests.

During Gregory's two years in office, many years of nursing experience were lost, and there is a strong argument to connect this loss to the stewardship of the new superintendent (SGHNDB). Several of those who left had long and unblemished records, but had either been disciplined immediately prior to their departure, for acts of insubordination, or were accused of poor performance. Whether Gregory was behaving in an overly autocratic way – in an attempt to gain control – or the head nurses were exploiting a perceived weakness in their new superintendent, the relation-ship does not seem to have been harmonious (SGHNDB).

This relationship was always a delicate balance. An inexperienced new superintendent (such as Gregory) was likely to encounter strong resistance from more experienced, older head nurses – especially if she attempted to interfere with established routines. Head nurses, accustomed to running their wards virtually unsupervised – answerable to the medical officers rather than the Matron – were threatened by the arrival of new-style super-intendents who challenged this autonomy. Miss Burt, Matron at Guy's in the 1880s, is a case in point. Trained by the St Johns' House Sisterhood, and with experience at several large hospitals, her appointment at Guy's caused great disruption among both the medical and nursing staff. The previous Matron, Mary Loag, had held the post since 1845 and many of her senior nurses had served similar lengths of time. Twenty Guy's nurses resigned in protest against the reforms Burt introduced (Waddington 1995; Moore 1988; Young 2008).

A similar breakdown in trust occurred at the Hospital for Sick Children at Great Ormond Street (HSC), in 1877, when the departure of its Lady Superintendent, Miss Dalrymple Hay, was followed by the resignation of all the sisters, out of loyalty to her and disapproval of her chosen successor.[13] Although all but one were persuaded to stay, their relationship with the new superintendent quickly soured, and after a year Mrs Dickin herself resigned, stating 'I feel strongly that my position here, is that of Lady Superintendent in name only, the control and superintendence being assumed by the "Sisters".' Her use of quotation marks suggests what she really thought of the voluntary, untrained ladies who constituted her staff (GOS/1/2/15, 22 November 1877).

Once established the bond between a superintendent and her head nurses could be strong, and cause as many problems as a poor relation-ship. That which existed between Miss Dalymple Hay and her sisters obviously fell into this category; as did that between the nurses and matron of the Sheffield Nurses' Home, a private nursing institution. Here, the entire nursing staff went on strike when their matron was forced to resign after complaining about overcrowding in the nurses' accommodation. She went on to found her own nurses' institution and many from the Sheffield Home joined her, leaving the original institution in crisis (*NR*, 31 May 1888: 101).[14]

It was not just lack of experience and association with an unpopular regime which caused Gregory's problems at St George's; class tensions probably also played a part. As a 'lady nurse', she was of superior social standing to her head nurses and this could have been a further cause of conflict.[15] The existence of class tensions within nursing has been docu-mented by historians; and the nursing journals, especially *The Hospital*, were full of letters on the subject (Abel-Smith 1960; Parry and Parry 1976).[16] On Gregory's resignation, the hospital appeared to lose faith in lady superintendents. They elected instead an older woman, with years of nursing experience and, most significantly, from a similar background to the head nurses. In Mrs Coster, the Board was perhaps looking for a steadying influence, after the unsettling experiment with 'modern' nurses.

Stability among the head nurses was eventually re-established. With other problems resolved, long service among this group probably became self-sustaining. Being working-class or lower-middle-class women (as discussed in Chapter 2), it is highly unlikely that they had independent means, and would therefore need to support themselves through work. As head nurses in a prestigious institution, they had attained a degree of financial security and a pension for their retirement. Why would they consider leaving? Further promotion opportunities outside the hospital rarely arose, and at St George's they had established reputations in a hospital which valued their contribution.

For those who did aspire to the post of matron, there was a short window of opportunity, when a woman had accumulated enough experience to inspire confidence, but was not in danger of being considered too old. Analysis of length of service of those who left St George's to become matrons suggests they had held their senior post for just under five years.[17] Taking training and ward experience into account, this suggests an optimum age to apply for a matron's job was in the early to mid-thirties; after that the likelihood of obtaining a top job began to wane.[18] Martha Vicinus has identified a similar preference for young leaders in other Victorian middle-class female occupations, such as teaching, which she assigned to a dearth of suitably qualified candidates, at least in the early days (1985). A similar argument can also be applied to nursing when 'modern nursing' was in its infancy, and middle-class candidates for higher posts were in relatively short supply.

In nursing, youth was prized because of the physically demanding nature of the work. The role of Matron (or Lady Superintendent, to situate this discussion in the 'new nursing system') required experience, but also demanded the energy and enthusiasms of youth. Well-known examples of longevity in the role exist (Miss Luckes at the London being a prime example) but there were also many whose careers were cut short through ill health.[19]

The trend for very young matrons emerged in the 1880s, when several influential hospitals appointed women in their mid-twenties. Eva Luckes became Matron at the London at the age of 26, while Ethel Manson (later, Ethel Fenwick) was appointed to St Bartholomew's when she was only 24 (McGann 1992). By the late 1880s, as standards of nurse education improved, it would have been impossible for similarly young, inexperienced women to manage a nursing department on sheer enthusiasm and energy alone, faced, as they would be, by an increasingly skilled workforce. A woman in her mid-thirties, who offered a balance of still youthful energy and good nursing experience, was therefore preferable.[20]

Matron posts became vacant rarely, and for most long-serving head nurses at St George's (of which there were many) the opportunity to rise to this position was no more than a distant dream. Still, they should not be considered as lacking in ambition, or inferior to their colleagues who aspired to higher things. Such women were comfortable in their roles, knew their doctors and managers well, and formed the backbone of an efficient nursing department. They were highly respected by superiors and their contribution to the running of the hospital was acknowledged.

Thomas Whipham, medical officer at the hospital in 1880, wrote of one head nurse: 'I have ... very considerable pleasure in calling your attention to some excellent work done by Head Nurse Moseley last week' (SGHNR/2 Moseley).[21]

Clinton Dent (surgeon and nurse lecturer at the hospital) had fulsome praise for Head Nurse Roberts:

> Nurse Roberts, while in nursing charge of my patient ... in the special ward displayed most commendable zeal and energy throughout ... [and] good judgement and much sagacity ... I think good nursing had much to do with weighing down the balance in the favourable direction.
>
> (SGHNR/3 Roberts)[22]

Dr Dunkin (another doctor on the staff) wrote of his approval at the appointment of Martha Reader to head nurse on his ward:

> I consider Miss Reader a very satisfactory nurse, and looking at the time she has had in which to obtain special skill in obstetrical work, a very promising one. I shall be quite satisfied ... with her in Wright Ward.
>
> (SGHNR/3 Reader)

Although the arrival of Mrs Coster appeared to quieten the unsettled head nurses, the poor retention of regular nurses was not resolved. Instability in the Department persisted throughout 1870s, as Figures 4.1 and 4.2 indicate, and was further threatened by difficulties in recruitment. The managers had to look for other causes of, and solutions to, the problem.

'Treat your good nurses well'

All was not well at St George's long before the crisis of 1872. In 1864, a special committee was formed to review nursing in the hospital, including wages and roles (SGHWB/33, 20 April 1864). It found there was increasing difficulty in hiring 'trustworthy and respectable nurses', and that in order to improve the situation, attention was needed to the conditions under which they served. It was necessary to 'treat the good nurses well', in terms of both remuneration and 'reasonable indulgences' (SGHWB/33, 27 April 1864). This was the first time managers had paid such attention to their nurses, and arguably marks the turning point in their view of nurses, from easily replaceable domestics to valuable assets. The committee prescribed an overhaul of pay scales, recommending annual pay rises (of £1 a year up to a maximum of £40) and a one-off gratuity payment – equivalent to 1.5–3 months' wages – for their most experienced head nurses. The package represented an wage increase of approximately 40 per cent, a great incentive to remain loyal to the hospital (SGHWB/33, 27 April 1864).

No similar review was recommended for assistant nurses. They had to wait until 1869, when the newly formed Committee of Nursing recommended their pay be increased from £18 to £20 to improve recruitment (SGHCON/1, 25 October 1869). This was an expensive move for an institution which operated on a financial knife-edge and to fund it the committee proposed radical measures with regard to nurses' overall conditions of employment.[23] Payment of board wages was to be suspended. Up to this point, although nurses lived in, they were paid £18 a year (in addition to their salary) for meals, refreshments and washing. In future these would be provided by the hospital directly (SGHCON/1, 29 March 1869). A uniform was also introduced and nurses were supplied with material to make up into dresses, caps and aprons, to a standard design (SGHCON/1, 6 February 1869).

The head nurses objected strenuously, particularly as a significant portion of their disposable income had been removed. They confronted the Committee of Nursing with their grievances, Head Nurse Robertson subsequently being censured for her manner in addressing them (SGHCON/1, 8 November 1869). The nurses were unsuccessful. Despite their objections (and previous pledges to treat nurses well), financial considerations took precedence. The changes in board arrangements were implemented, and saved £216 a year, the savings being used to fund the assistant nurses' pay rise and the material for uniforms (SGHWB/35, 3 November 1869). In a further challenge to head nurses' loyalty, their maximum wage was reduced from £40 to £35 a year (SGHCON/1 25 October 1869).[24] How this affected the relationship between head nurses and assistant nurses was not recorded.

Thereafter, nurse wages were reviewed regularly, as illustrated in Figure 4.3. In 1874, aware of competition for nurse recruits posed by other hospitals, the managers carried out a survey of nurses' wages in London. It must have revealed a significant disparity, as wages at St George's rose again (SGHCON/1, 7 December 1874).

The pressure to review wages sometimes came from the nurses themselves, who were not afraid to make their own case to the Board. In 1852, the head nurses presented a written petition to the Weekly Board, demanding wages be reviewed in the light of a recent increase awarded to night nurses:

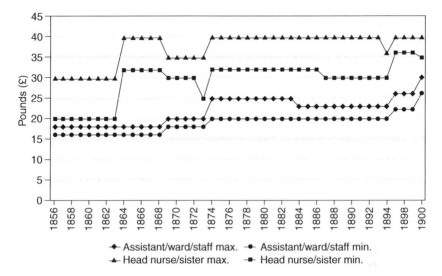

Figure 4.3 Evolution of nurses' wages at St George's, 1856–1900 (sources: 1853–99 St George's Hospital Weekly Board Minutes; 1868–99 St George's Hospital Committee of Nursing Minutes. St George's Hospital Nurses' Wage Book, 1849–60.)

We the undersigned ... beg [to address you] in relation to our duties and salary, and as much as you have very kindly considered those of the night nurses, whose duties are much less arduous than ours, we do hope that you will kindly consider our case.

(SGHWB/28, 9 February 1853)

They were called before the Board to be told their case would receive attention; and the following week a new salary scale for head nurses was announced (SGHWB/28, 16 February 1853).

Even probationers were prepared to fight against perceived injustices. In 1895, second-year probationers sent a petition to the Committee of Nursing in which they complained about changes to their pay. They were angered by a recent decision, introduced during their first year, to halt the practice of promoting the best second-year probationers to ward nurses (with the corresponding increase in salary), thus leaving them out of pocket. In response, the committee acknowledged the confusion and offered those affected a gratuity of £4, if they completed their second year successfully (SGHCON/2, 11 March 1895).

The determination of St George's nurses to have some control over their lives shows through in these examples; as does their confidence to stand up to the all-male management committees, to demand just and fair treatment.

Martha Vicinus has claimed that, unlike other female institutions such as women's colleges, sisterhoods and settlements, nursing did not develop the same feeling of community among its members. She characterizes nursing departments as hierarchical organizations dominated by one woman, at odds with their medical colleagues, and with each other (1985). This lack of cohesion was also remarked upon at the time. Dr Bedford Fenwick wrote of the 'lamentable deficiency of *esprit de corps* amongst Nurses', which he assigned to 'the want of organization' or 'the strange inability of women to work with other women to a common end' (*NR*, 24 September 1891: 158).

The view of a profession at odds with itself is perpetuated by modern historians' focus on the battles over nurse registration and accusations of snobbery in nursing which set middle-class nurses against their lower-class colleagues (Witz 1992). The penchant for establishing rival organizations, from which to heap heavy criticism on the opposition, does not engender a view of a unified community. Neither do the reams of letters published in the nursing journals from 'Lady Nurses' condemning their 'servant class' colleagues, or the latter who accuse 'ladies' of stealing their livelihoods.[25]

However, this very public and political rivalry between two warring factions may not be reflective of the body of nursing. The nurses at St George's demonstrated their community cohesion in joint petitions to managers over holidays, uniforms and changes to duties, as well as wages. Neither did they restrict communal action to self-interest: they also acted together on behalf of hospital servants, on one occasion causing disquiet among the managers when they organized a Christmas collection for dining-hall staff (SHGCON/2 30 November 1896).[26] These nurses – able to stand up for themselves, and others, against the might of male official-dom – present a vivid contrast to the traditional image of the Victorian nurse as docile, obedient and meek, and cast doubt on Vicinus' claim that they lacked a sense of community (Maggs 1980; Peterson 1989; Vickery 1998).

The Weekly Board used nurses' wages as both an incentive for recruit-ment and an inducement to stay. The gap between minimum and maximum wages for all levels represented the potential for annual pay rises, regardless of opportunities for promotion. Wages generally increased by £1 a year, if performance was satisfactory, until the maximum was reached; thus good behaviour was rewarded and prolonged service encouraged.[27] Even a probationer's meagre wages rose for each year of training, though she was contractually bound to serve a minimum number of years. On successful completion of training, and promotion to ward nurse, a probationer could expect a further two to five years of pay rises, taking her well beyond her contracted time. Inducements to head nurses continued for even longer, generally holding the promise of additional income for a period of at least five years. If the tactic was successful, the managers would realize their goal of a Nursing Department staffed by nurses trained within the hospital, with a gratifying level of experience between them.

Despite regularly checking its wages against other London hospitals, the Board paid no attention to those in other employment sectors. Although women's work opportunities had widened considerably by the end of the nineteenth century, the absence of comparison with other occupations suggests that they were not considered to be direct competitors for recruits. By the beginning of the 1890s, nursing had become heavily oversubscribed, and the main competition for the best recruits came from other hospitals.[28]

'An absolute luxury ... every nurse her own bedroom'

While wages were an important part of the package to recruit and retain nurses, there was also the matter of 'reasonable indulgences', designed to make a nurse's life a little more tolerable (SGHWB/33, 27 April 1864). The parlous state of their accommodation was identified repeatedly as a contributing factor to retention problems. As early as 1858, the Board was so concerned about recurring complaints that it commissioned a wide-ranging review of nurses' quarters.

The final report was damning: 'exceedingly defective and totally inadequate', was how the sleeping accommodation was described (SGHWB/30, 1 December 1858). Forty-eight nurses slept in 21 rooms, with 'only 657 cubic feet' per nurse. Some rooms were only six feet high. Only eight had chimneys, but only five of these had grates and therefore a place to cook meals or keep a fire in winter. The remaining rooms had no such luxury. In two, which housed eight nurses between them, there were no fireplaces or external windows; the only ventilation or source of natural light came from two vents opening onto a stairwell. Other rooms had sky lights or 'borrowed lights'; and through some of them, 'small and unventilated as they are, the pipes containing hot water for the warming of the hospital pass'. The pipes might have provided a welcome source of heat in winter, but in the absence of ventilation could have made cramped rooms insufferably warm. With no kitchen facilities, and no grates in their bedrooms, meals were cooked on ward fires. Rats were a common problem, some rooms suffered badly from damp and others from noxious fumes from nearby water closets (SGHWB/28, 16 and 23 March 1853; SGHWB/30, 1 December 1858).

Immediate remedial action was ordered, to provide a minimum of 1,000 cubic feet per nurse, individual bedrooms for head nurses, and appropriate cooking facilities for all. Plans were drawn up for the accommodation to be constructed on the roof. The new facilities, which opened in November 1859, provided separate accommodation for the night staff (protecting them from disturbance by their daytime colleagues), single

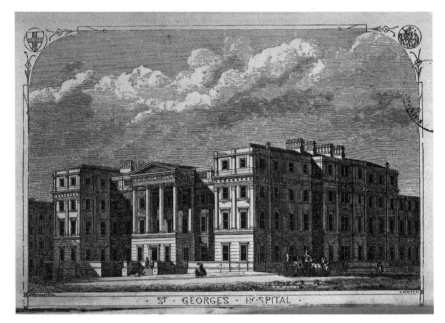

Plate 2 Exterior of St George's Hospital, *c.*1859. © *Country Life.* Reproduced courtesy of St George's Hospital Medical School Library.

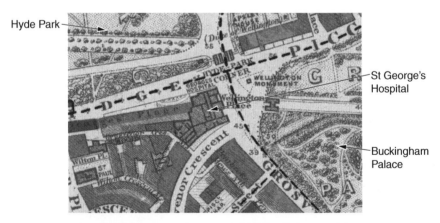

Plate 3 St George's Hospital and environs, 1898–9. Charles Booth Poverty Maps. Reproduced courtesy of the Library of the London School of Economics and Political Science.

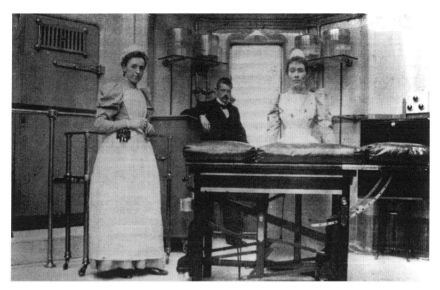

Plate 4 Nurses in one of the operating theatres at St George's, *c.*1898 (with Dr Lloyd, as a student, in the background). Courtesy of St George's Hospital Medical School Library.

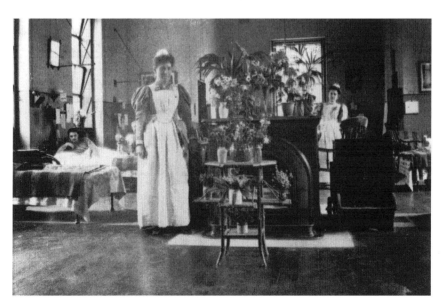

Plate 5 Nurses in Belgrave Ward, St George's, *c.*1898. Courtesy of St George's Hospital Medical School Library.

rooms for eight head nurses and three new rooms to accommodate nine assistant nurses. (Plate 2, p. 124, shows the exterior of hospital after the new floor had been completed.) All rooms had windows and fireplaces; a scullery, kitchen and water closet were also built.

The new accommodation represented a significant improvement, but a number of nurses were still sleeping in the main hospital, leaving them open to the 'hospital atmosphere' (SGHWB/31, 26 October 1859). Their living quarters continued to be a source of concern. In 1863, a visitor reported that the 'Nurse's room of Hope Ward is frequently offensive from the water closets of nearby Ratcliffe Ward' (SGHWB/32, 28 October 1863). In 1870, the Night Superintendent's wooden bedstead had to be replaced, being 'very much overrun with vermin', and later the same year the Apothecary condemned several assistant nurses' bedrooms as unfit for habitation (SGHCON/1, 28 February 1870, 29 July 1870 and 28 November 1870). A year later, the rooms of four head nurses – which opened directly onto their wards – were reportedly without doors, depriving their occupants of privacy and leaving them exposed to the hospital's dangerous miasmas. Doors were ordered to be fitted immediately, to keep out 'the foul air from the ward' (SGHCON/1, 3 October 1871).

Nurses continued to sleep several to a room, sometimes with curtain partitions to provide a modicum of privacy. The rooms were candlelit and unheated, except in instances of extreme cold (SHGWB/57, 21 November 1894).[29]

Zepharina Veitch made the connection between recruitment and accommodation in one of her first proposals on joining the hospital. The installation of communal dining and relaxation areas, she claimed, would go a long way to addressing the 'comfort and improvement of the nurses [making it] easier ... to secure a superior class of women for the work' (SGHCON/1, 1 March 1869). Provision of such luxuries, still a rarity at any London hospital, would confer great advantage in the competition for good quality recruits. Veitch's plans were not implemented entirely: lack of space was the proverbial problem. A communal dining area was established, but the sitting room could not be accommodated. Nearly ten years later the idea was still being mooted, the Committee for Nursing lamenting that such a facility would 'add much to [the] comfort [of nurses]', even if it would not resolve the immediate problem of staff retention (SGHCON/1, 12 March 1877).

By 1885 progress had been made on several fronts. The hospital's Annual Report praised the quality of nurse accommodation now available:

> The Board have long felt that in order to induce a better class of persons to offer themselves as nurses they must improve the accommodation for them in the hospital, and have at last completed certain alterations which greatly add to their comfort. In the past it was usual for [nurses] to sleep two or even three to a room, but now each nurse

has a separate sleeping apartment and in addition to a good dining room there is a well furnished sitting room open for those off duty.

(SGHAR 1885)

It is clear that the standard of accommodation was seen as key to attracting superior candidates to the Nursing Department, and that the hospital was prepared to go to some lengths to achieve this. Most London hospitals had to grapple with the problem of nurse accommodation. In 1886, Eva Luckes persuaded the London Hospital Board, against much opposition, to provide separate bedrooms for her nurses, in addition to dining and sitting rooms. Ethel Fenwick also campaigned for better nurse accommodation at St Bartholomew's (McGann 1992). But it was always a battle with the joint obstacles of finance and space.

New nurse accommodation was included in expansion plans at St George's throughout the rest of the century, and was constructed whenever space and funds allowed. Nevertheless, lack of accommodation was often the main reason for rejecting proposals to extend the Nursing Department. Availability of space was in danger of dictating the quality of nursing. In 1890, a further influx of nurses prompted a major accommodation crisis. Plans were drawn up to redevelop the hospital's entire central block, adding new operating theatres and additional accommodation for both nurses and resident doctors; but estimates came in at £65,000, and the ideas were rejected (SGHWB/53, 13 June 1890).

Continual reorganization of the existing space over the years had resulted in nurse accommodation being spread throughout the hospital buildings. For several years, the nurses' recreation room was at the top of the hospital (fashioned out of the old convalescent ward) while the dining room was in the basement. Sleeping rooms were scattered anywhere in between, often crammed in stairwells, over operating theatres, next to water closets and sculleries. As a result, the accommodation bore a closer resemblance to servants' quarters than the type of apartment familiar to the young middle-class women the hospital was trying to attract. The logical solution would have been a comprehensive programme of renovation of nurse accommodation; but such a scheme required money and space. Both were in short supply at all central London hospitals, which had grown organically around their original eighteenth-century buildings. St George's location posed a particular challenge. Hemmed in by the houses of London's upper classes, royal parks and palaces, there was no space for development, apart from up (see Plate 3, p. 124). When the 1890 plans were rejected, there was no alternative but to move nurse accommodation off site.

St George's had neither paying probationers nor a private nursing institute to fund the purchase of adjacent buildings – which, given the socio-economic profile of its neighbourhood, would have been prohibitively expensive anyway. It did have an extensive property portfolio, however, and finally lighted on a terrace of houses in Montpelier Street, Chelsea, as the location for its new nurses' home.

The scheme did not meet with unanimous approval (SGHWB/53 18 June 1890; SGHCON/2 1 December 1890). Objections raised, most notably by the Chairman of the Committee of Nursing, Hugh Macpherson, illustrate the paternalistic attitude adopted by hospital officials towards their nurses. Nurses could not be properly managed, Macpherson argued, if they were at such a distance from the main hospital – implying the need for constant supervision (SGHCON/2, 1 December 1890). He felt so strongly on the subject that he resigned; but despite his resignation, the move went ahead. The new home opened in 1892, providing, 'very comfortable accommodation for twenty-three nurses' (SGHWB/54 13 April 1892). By 1895, however, shoddy workmanship (the result of cost-cutting in the original conversion) was revealed in an architect's report: 'Roofs are in a shaky state and have been strutted up and repaired frequently ... rain has come into the brickwork which on the upper floors is much decayed ... floors are sagging and have been frequently patched' (SGHWB/57, 6 February 1895). The nurses' home no longer sounded quite so comfortable. The only feasible recourse was to demolish the whole terrace and erect a new purpose-built home on the site, and this time the Quarterly Court had no option. Building work was sanctioned (SGHWB/57, 8 February 1895).

The work was actually financed by a generous supporter, and the the Major Charles Hall Memorial Home for Nurses opened in 1897, to great fanfare (SGHWB/58, 6 January 1897; SGHAR 1896). It accommodated 80 nurses in single rooms, and provided a dining room, sitting room, writing room and garden. Each bedroom had a fireplace, and electric lighting was used throughout. Rooms at Montpelier Street must have been jealously coveted by those who remained at the hospital. Their rooms were still lit by candlelight, and there was no outside space to compare with the garden at the new home. To temper these disadvantages, a new nurses' sitting room with a 'magnificent view over Hyde Park' was opened; and the reduction in numbers at the hospital meant each nurse could at last have her own room. Matron Smedley described the accommodation as, 'an absolute luxury for every nurse to have her own bedroom instead of a cubicle' (*H/NM*, 18 November 1899).

The Weekly Board – by introducing sitting rooms, library and piano – was attempting the difficult task of recreating a middle-class retreat in the midst of the hospital (SGHCON/1, 13 June 1881; SGHWB/47, 4 April 1883). The same strategy was used by other organizations hoping to attract middle-class women. Schools for young women, such as Cheltenham Ladies College – and university colleges, such as Newnham and Girton at Cambridge and Somerville at Oxford – strove to create a middle-class family environment within their institutions (M.B. Vickery 2000). Emily Davies, founder of Girton, chose an existing house for her new college because the alternative (a new building fashioned along the lines of men's colleges) afforded too many unsupervised areas. A house, with its communal dining and sitting rooms, 'encouraged community' and made surveillance easier (M.B. Vickery 2000). Such measures addressed the dual needs of reassuring parents that their daughters were safe, and providing familiar surroundings to young women leaving the protection of their families for the first time (Dyhouse 1981; Adams 1996; Pedersen 2002).

Large department stores – which employed young middle-class women in growing numbers towards the end of the century – also attempted to attract applicants by providing comfortable facilities. Lady shopworkers at Howell & James of Regent Street were offered separate bedrooms, a sitting room, library and a piano (Grogan 1880).[30] Even non-residential workers were provided with a familiar environment. The Prudential offered its lady clerks a library, a piano, a luncheon room and a terrace, reached by a staircase to which male clerks had no access (Davin 2005).

The challenges of attracting middle-class women into hospitals, populated as they were by the morally suspect working classes, were even tougher. What parent could be entirely comfortable with their impressionable young daughter working and living in the midst of a working-class enclave? The accommodation hospitals aspired to provide should therefore be as separate as possible from the working-class maelstrom (while maintaining efficiency in running the wards), and replicate the middle-class home (Jordan 1999). Financial and physical difficulties often conspired against these ideals.

Ann Simnet has suggested that the creation of middle-class culture within nursing served an alternative purpose, to drive away working-class women (1986). These women, she claims, would have found the culture intimidating, preferring instead more familiar surroundings, such as factories. Recruitment at St George's does not support this. Working-class women continued to join the hospital as nurses, arguably attracted precisely because of the emerging middle-class culture, and associated opportunities for social advancement.[31]

'Reasonable indulgences'[32]

Nurses' leave arrangements also came under review in the Board's quest to attract and retain good nurses. Annual holidays for regular nurses rose from one week in the 1850s to three weeks by the end of the century, while head nurses' leave increased from one week to four over the same period. Monthly and weekly leave also increased and as did the number of hours off-duty during the day (SGH Archive).

Annual breaks from the daily routine acquired new importance in the Victorian psyche. In 1869, *The Standard* described the annual holiday as, 'a good and wholesome practice' enjoyed by everyone from 'the heir to the throne to the humblest greengrocer' (quoted in Horn 1999: 122). Thirty years later, the *Fortnightly Review* declared that annual holidays were no longer the 'luxury of the wealthy, but a necessity of the workers as much ... [as] food and clothing' (quoted in Horn 1999: 122). Growth in the railways, both at home and on the continent, offered urban residents easy and relatively cheap access to the seaside, and made travel across Europe economically more feasible. Thomas Cook's company, established mid-century, shuttled middle-class tourists around the globe in the first wave of mass foreign tourism (Thompson 1988: 262–3). In the 1880s, mill workers in Lancashire 'streamed off to the seaside by train' for their newly won holidays; while railway companies introduced paid breaks for their workers in the 1870s, a privilege also enjoyed by clerks in local and central government (Thompson 1988: 276). For those whose financial situation precluded a whole week away, day trips offered a chance to escape for a few hours. Whatever the choice, families saved 'strenuously ... and spent lavishly' on their holiday activity (Best 1979 [1985]).

Nurses were no exception. By the early 1890s most (especially those in institutions) had some form of annual leave. Letters in the nursing journals contained advice on how to spend this time. Some visited family, especially if they lived at some distance from their place of work. However, those with no family or friends to visit were left to make their own arrangements from 'resources [which are] very limited' (*NR*, 6 July 1895: 495). One writer suggested that the Royal British Nurses' Association (RBNA) should establish a 'Nurses' Cooperative Travel' to help those who wanted a holiday, but lacked funds or companions. Similar initiatives, by the Polytechnic at Regent Street and the Home Reading Union, had proved very popular.[33]

A scheme to provide nurses with rest and recuperation in the country was set up by Philippa Hicks, a sister at King's College Hospital.[34] She persuaded personal friends take nurses for a short stay in their country homes. The scheme received support from luminaries such as Henry Burdett:

> [It] has proved a great success ... worthy of generous support. The plan has been tried for some years and has proved so great a boon to the nurses ... that ... its extension by getting more ladies to offer a fortnight's change to those who need it [is desirable].
>
> (Burdett 1890: 136)

Burdett believed it was important for nurses to 'get away from the shop' (Burdett 1890: 135). Staying in the house of a lady, where a nurse could escape the evil humours of a hospital, but where her behaviour could still be monitored, was probably an ideal arrangement. Hicks offered to fund a network of 'homes of rest' for holidaying nurses, but her offer received mixed response. While Burdett and the like lavished praise on the scheme, nurses were sceptical. What they needed most was a break from institutional life and an escape from the company of other nurses (*H/NM*, 4 April 1888: 25). Better to increase nurses' pay, they argued, so they could support themselves on holiday, rather than depend on charitable homes; and far from 'homes of rest', they wanted a complete change in environment, to pursue active pastimes, such as cycling, boating, tennis and riding (*H/NM*, 14 June 1890: xliii).

Nurses wrote to the journals advertising for travelling companions and exchanging ideas, although from the costs involved, most must have had independent means. One invited nurses to join her on a trip to Switzerland. It would last a month and cost in the region of £15 (*H/NM*, 25 June 1892). As this was equivalent to nearly half the wages of a head nurse at St George's, its cost would preclude regular hospital nurses from participating.[35] But nurses with less disposable income (or time) had options. A lady in Cheshire offered accommodation from five shillings a week, which, with a train fare of 29 shillings, would have created a two-week holiday for just over £2 (*H/NM*, 21 July 1894). This was much more affordable. A visit to the coast was also possible: accommodation could be had in Southend, for instance, for 30 shillings a week with a train fare from London of only two shillings (*H/NM*, 21 July 1894).

Activity-based holidays were also popular. One writer described the delights of a walking tour; while another was ambivalent on the merits of golf. The advantages of being in the fresh air and sun all day were indisputable; but she was concerned that any benefits may be countered by an eruption of 'golf fever', which left participants exhausted by the strain of 'everlasting putting' (*H/NM*, 14 May 1892; *NR*, 31 October 1896: 367).

Annual leave was used as an incentive to retain nurses in much the same way as pay reviews, by linking leave entitlement to length of service. In one initiative, all nurses of at least three years' service were given an additional day's holiday for each year worked, up to maximum of seven extra days (SGHCON/2, 11 January 1892). A separate scheme, aimed at newly qualified probationers, awarded one month's leave at the end of training to those who had obtained staff positions – on condition that they returned to work for a contracted length of time (SGHCON/2, 12 January 1891). For a probationer, accustomed to one week's annual leave in total, this could have been a strong incentive to sign up for an additional period.[36]

As the importance of regular breaks became increasingly recognized, focus turned to the provision of daily leave, in addition to annual escapes. Burdett made a strong plea for more recreation time for nurses: 'They have been thought of as ministering angels', he wrote, 'but ... as angels who have few or no wants of their own ... who are able and willing to give all, asking nothing in return' (*H/NM*, 5 March 1887: 379).

Nurses were not angels, though, but human beings, and like fellow-women, they needed rest and recreation. In Burdett's (paternalistic) view, hospitals should provide diversions for its nurses: a programme of gymnastic exercise was one suggestion. If that was not feasible, singing and dancing would be a suitable substitute (*H/NM*, 5 March 1887).

Interest in physical exercise was reaching new heights. Therapeutic exercise was fashionable among middle-class women and medically pre-scribed gentle exercise, remedial gymnastics and massage were used to treat a wide range of female complaints (Hargreaves 2001). The London School Board introduced Swedish gymnastics in its elementary schools as early as 1878, and clubs for young women, such as the Polytechnic, offered physical training classes (Holcombe 1973). Against this background, it is not surprising that physical exercise should be recommended for nurses (Holcombe 1973). Burdett's interest in gymnastics may not have been confined to its physical benefits; he may also have seen an ideal opportun-ity to reinforce 'mechanical obedience', as it was used in the elementary schools (Holcombe 1973: 61).

The gymnasia and specialist trainers may not have materialized, but hospital managers (perhaps even more so than other employers) began to recognize the importance of daily time away from the wards. A few hours off the wards gave nurses a break in routine (itself considered beneficial) and an escape from the hospital atmosphere, heavy with infectious miasmas and decay. At St George's, head nurses were first granted daily leave, of two hours, in 1877 (SGHCON/1, 9 July 1877). The luxury was not extended to regular nurses until many years later, despite their frequent petitions for the privilege. The apparently insurmountable problem of providing cover for nurses on breaks ensured such requests were always rejected (SGHCON/2 10 July 1893). The matter came to a head, in 1894, after a survey showed daily leave to be the norm at other hospitals. One had responded,

> We have not seen anything like the number of small breakdowns that we had under the old system, and the work in the wards is better done because the Nurses are not working under the same pressure. Hours out of the Wards rest them more and send them back to their labours with a good store of strength, bright and cheerful and very fit for work.
>
> (SGHCON/2 7 May 1894)

The committee was forced into action, but once again, only after looking beyond its own walls. Daily leave of two hours was granted to every nurse.[37] The purpose of the new leave was made clear in a set of rules for proba-tioners published in 1898: they were entitled to 'two hours every day for *outdoor* recreation' (SGHCON/2 10 March 1898, my emphasis).

Advice to nurses on how to spend their daily leave abounded: outdoor pursuits, which removed nurses from the noxious fumes of the hospital, were strongly recommended:

Temptation to spend time off duty on a bed ... ought to be fought against as bad both for the mind and the body. The effort made to start for an entertainment is always repaid by weariness forgotten, whereas reposing on a sofa only keeps one in mind of one's tiredness.

(*H/NM*, 8 December 1888)

Following the middle-class predilection for uplifting or improving diversions, visits to museums or galleries, going for a walk, or attending the theatre or a concert were frequent recommendations. *Conversazione*, held by the large hospitals, provided nurses with a safe environment in which to meet friends and enjoy an evening's entertainment. The largest, and most lavish, was organized annually by the Royal British Nurses Association. Held at prestigious addresses in London, upwards of a 1,000 guests – including nurses, matrons and dignitaries – came from all over the country. The programme lasted for three hours, and included music and recitation from well-known entertainers of the day (*H/NM*, 15 December 1888).[38]

At St George's, medical officers, students and hospital supporters organized an annual event for nurses' entertainment; and in return, the nurses sang glees. The events took place in the hospital boardroom – a place more normally associated with reprimands than jollity. But, unlike Burdett, who exhorted hospitals to provide ever more activities and entertainments for its nurses, Smedley regarded her nurses as adults, capable of amusing themselves. Apart from the occasional concert, there were no other special arrangements in place (*H/NM*, 18 November 1899).

By the end of the century, nurses' homes were equipped with tennis courts, or had clubs for cycling or walking. The new home at Montpelier Street included a tennis court in the garden (SGHWB/54, 4 May 1892). Guy's nurses had their own cycling club, based at a cottage in Lewisham (*H/NM*, 12 September 1896), despite the controversy surrounding women and cycling.[39] One matron wrote to *The Hospital* that her nurses were banned from cycling, because of her personal feelings towards 'female cyclists' (*H/NM*, 1 October 1898). Support for this view flooded in, but equal numbers countered it. A private nurse wrote '[my] health is greatly benefited by ... rides', and she encouraged others to take up cycling as convenient method of travelling around (*NR*, 29 September 1900: 257). The plans for Montpelier Street had also included an entrance for bicycles in the basement, but this element was later removed. The decision was probably financial, rather than a desire to prohibit the use of bicycles. With the majority of its nurses now located at some distance from the hospital, it is likely that cycling to work would be encouraged, particularly as the Board had been obliged to pay nurses' bus fares (SGHWB/58, 18 November 1896; SHGCON/2, 18 January 1897).

A new system of nursing

Improvements in accommodation and leave entitlement were expected to ease problems of recruitment and retention, but further reforms were deemed necessary. In 1879, concerned that the hospital was falling behind other institutions, the Committee of Nursing reported:

> [being] driven to the consideration [of changes] owing to the great difficulty experienced of late in obtaining efficient persons as assistant nurses. These difficulties have been increased by the fact that, at other hospitals, the changes proposed have already been carried out.
>
> (SGHWB/43, 5 March 1879)

It was the nurses themselves who brought the central issue (the content of their role) to the attention of the Committee:

> [we] have more 'cleaning' duties to perform [at St George's] than at other Hospitals, & that [we] have so frequently to leave the ward for the purpose of fetching various things from the Kitchen, Dispensary, &c, that the strictly nursing duties which [we] are able to discharge are few in comparison, [our] office being rather that of a servant than of a trained nurse.
>
> (SGHWB/43, 5 March 1879)

The continued reliance on nurses to perform domestic chores discouraged suitably qualified women from joining the hospital, and obviously disenchanted the women who joined. As nurse training became more complex, it is not surprising that nurses began to view themselves as specialist workers, possessed of valuable skills. The continued inclusion of cleaning and scrubbing in their duties threatened this view and diluted its impact.[40] After further surveys of other hospitals, the managers bowed to nurses' demands, and ward servants were hired to relieve nurses of the heaviest chores. Once again, the impetus for change had come from comparison with other hospitals. The difference on this occasion was that St George's failure to keep pace was pointed out by the nurses themselves.

Considerable changes to the Nursing Department's structure were also introduced at this time. There was little opportunity for promotion in the existing structure, and for assistant nurses (who had no authority whatsoever) there was little chance for betterment. Such lack of prospects was identified as a major cause of poor retention. If the problem was to be overcome, changes in the distribution of the workload would have to be implemented. The number of head nurses was reduced, giving those who remained responsibility for groups of wards. They assumed supervisory, rather than day-to-day, management roles. Among other benefits, this gave head nurses more time to train probationers, whose numbers were steadily increasing (SGHWB/43 7 May 1879). Daily ward management was transferred to a new team of ward nurses (one to each ward), assisted by probationers. The assistant nurse post was abolished, replaced by the new ward nurse, and the despised scrubbing and heavy cleaning elements were removed from their remit (SGHWB/43, 7 May 1879).

Of course, the scheme encountered opposition from both medical and nursing staff. Neither the doctors nor nurses fully accepted the duties of the new 'ward nurse', and two years after its introduction, ward nurses had still not taken on all the responsibilities envisaged. The failure was assigned 'to reluctance on the part of old head nurses to delegate to the ward nurses duties they have done themselves for years' (SGHCON/1, 26 Jan 1880; SGHWB/45, 13 April 1881). The medical staff were also resistant, reluctant to 'receive reports and communicate their orders to the ward nurses', preferring to deal with the old head nurses with whom they were familiar (SGHWB/45, 13 April 1881).[41]

The reluctance of medical staff to accept new systems of nursing was commonplace (Waddington 1995). In the dispute at Guy's (discussed earlier) the medical staff and nurses reacted angrily to the introduction of a 'modern' matron. She threatened to upset their existing relationships by taking too much power into her own hands, challenging the authority of the doctors. The dispute was resolved only after the entire medical staff was threatened with dismissal (Waddington 1995). It received wide press coverage and caused a scandal for the hospital. Occurring contemporaneously with St George's own plans, Guy's problems must have given St George's managers and medics pause for thought. At Guy's, though, the Treasurer had acted unilaterally, but at St George's the medics had been consulted on all decisions: both through the Medical School Committee and the Committee of Nursing. Having been complicit in its conception, the doctors at St George's were in no position to challenge the new system of nursing outright.

Cumulatively, the changes appeared to have an immediate effect on both recruitment and retention of regular nurses. The annual report on nursing for 1880 stated, for the first time, that there had been no difficulty in maintaining a full staff of ward nurses, and, 'we continue to get a better class of candidates than formerly' (SGHWB/45, 13 April 1881). With more stability in the Nursing Department, a second objective was also now achievable. In the same report, the committee stated that for the first time since the policy was introduced over 25 years earlier, all head nurse vacancies had been filled internally (SGHWB/45, 13 April 1881).

A career in nursing at St George's?

A clear career path within the Nursing Department emerged as a result of these reforms. The best probationers became ward nurses, and were encouraged to remain with incentives such as regular wage increases and additional leave. As ward nurses, they were no longer at the bottom of the pile, but had responsibility for an entire ward; and with appropriate amount of experience, the best were appointed as supernumerary head nurses, until a vacancy arose. As the hospital grew and medicine evolved, new specialist nursing roles, such as theatre nurse and out patients' nurse, appeared. Judging by their wages, they were placed above ward nurse in the hospital hierarchy and offered additional opportunities for career development.[42]

Other hospitals had identified the benefits of a well-defined career path for their nurses. As early as 1871, St Mary's operated a system of nursing, 'features of which are not to be found elsewhere', whereby sisters were promoted from the body of nurses. The promise of progression was found to be 'highly motivating' for the nursing staff (*The Lancet*, 30 December 1871: 929).

But the idea of internal promotion was not universally accepted. Hospitals which maintained a two-tier, class-based nursing department – such as St Thomas', the London or King's – restricted entry to senior posts to women from superior social backgrounds (Booth, interviews with matrons, B153 1896). At other hospitals, promotion from the ranks was equally difficult, but for different reasons. Katharine Lumsden (Superintendent at the Aberdeen Sick Children's Hospital) argued against the promotion of nurses from within the same institution, using military analogy so favoured of some nurse leaders:

> To promote a non-commissioned officer in his own regiment is, unless he is endowed with exceptional tact and judgement, to place him in an awkward and difficult position, and the same objection holds good, I should think, in the case of a Hospital Nurse.
>
> (Lumsden 1896: 242)

When Florence Smedley was appointed Matron at St George's, she immediately reversed the internal recruitment policy. Her experience at the HSC (which adhered to Lumsden's view of internal promotion) may have influenced her decision, although it is also possible that she simply found the standard of nurse training at St George's (and therefore its nurses) did not meet her needs.[43]

However, up to this point, internal recruitment was adhered to and few head nurses were recruited externally. The managers hoped this made St George's an attractive place to train. But the policy was double-edged. Promotion to head nurse may have been possible, but increasing stability within the Department reduced the frequency with which vacancies arose.

Above that rank, opportunities were even rarer; the very ambitious had to look elsewhere to further their careers. At the other end of the scale there were also problems. With more stability generally, and an escalating number of probationers, the hospital was producing more trained nurses than it needed. This was not bad planning – it was beneficial in several aspects. The hospital could pick the very best trainees to fill staff nurse posts; while the large staff of probationers provided a cheap workforce. Rejected probationers must have been frustrated, and there is evidence that some tried to hang on to their posts for as long as possible.[44] However, even if a job at St George's did not materialize, most left with a certificate of training which would open up a wide range of opportunities.

The problem faced by probationers is illustrated in Figure 4.4. In the 1880s, 80 per cent were retained by the hospital, but by the 1890s nearly 50 per cent failed to find a job in the hospital. Of those who did, the majority never progressed beyond the rank of ward nurse. The odds were stacked against them: in 1894 there were 65 probationers on staff but only 21 head nurses and 34 ward nurses. With head nurses serving between five and seven years on average, vacancies were slow to materialize. Fewer than 10 per cent of probationers achieved this lofty position.

Competition for these posts must have been fierce, and the situation was exacerbated by Smedley's abandonment of internal recruitment. In her first two years, she recruited six sisters externally.[45] The editor of *St George's Hospital Gazette* (the Medical School's journal) criticized her policy:

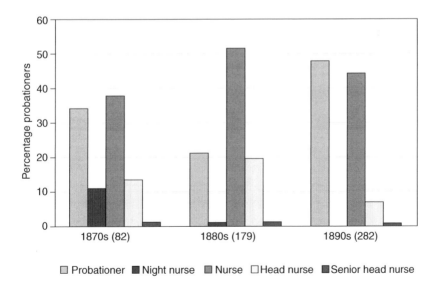

Figure 4.4 Careers of probationers at St George's (sources: St George's Hospital Nurses' Database, 1840–1900).

General surprise and no little heart burning has been caused by the fact that the vacant posts have been filled by Sisters from other hospitals ... We have Supernumerary Sisters trained at our own Hospital, any of whom in our humble opinion, are quite competent to take charge of a ward.

(*St George's Hospital Gazette*, June 1898)

The change in recruitment policy generated controversy outside the hospital. Ever willing take up the nurses' cause against the medical men, the *Nursing Record* rebuked the editor of the *Gazette*. 'We receive his opinion as to the suitability of candidates [as] sisters with about the same amount of respect as he would ours [for] house surgeons' (*NR*, 11 June 1898: 470). Medical students might have been happy with 'competent' nurses, but it seems Smedley's sights were set higher.

The Committee of Nursing hesitated over external recruitment, commenting more than once that such measures were only temporary (SGHCON/2, 13 November 1898). But they were in thrall to their new matron, who bombarded them (in a manner reminiscent of Zepharina Veitch) with a series of reforms affecting every aspect of nursing: mostly, she was successful. Many of her ideas originated from her time at the HSC, including the establishment of a contributory nurse pension scheme, the introduction of a structured curriculum for probationers, and her ideas on external recruitment. As the *Nursing Record* reported, on her retirement in 1907, 'when she took up her duties ... many urgent reforms were necessary to bring the Nursing Department up to date' (*NR*, 26 October 1907: 333). In only three years, Smedley had transformed the Nursing Department rendering it almost unrecognizable from the days of Harriet Coster.

Conclusion

Between 1870 and 1900, the managers of St George's Hospital adopted strategies to enhance its attractiveness to potential recruits, and to stop the revolving door through which nurses came and went at rapid rate. They were painfully aware of the competitive nature of nurse recruitment in the capital, and carried out numerous surveys of practice at other hospitals on topics as diverse as wages, leave entitlement and standard of accommodation. Policies on nursing were developed with one eye on public perception as it was increasingly recognized that the Nursing Department was the hospital's most public face, with significant potential to affect its image and ability to raise funds. As Clinton Dent commented:

[The nurses] became an essential element in the organization ... the reputation of the Hospital was given to a great extent into their keeping: what they did well they did for the good of the House; and what they did badly reflected ill on the institution as a whole.

(Dent 1894c)

The comfort of the nurses became a focus of the managers' attention as never before. When the improvements to their living conditions are viewed together, a picture emerges of efforts to create a more middle-class environment within the hospital – or as close to a middle-class home as was feasible in a vast and rambling institution. Improvements to accommodation and facilities, the staging of soirées and slide shows as entertainment, discussions of tennis courts and bicycle parks, all contribute to this middle-class image, to which the hospital aspired for its nurses.

The impetus for these changes came mainly as a result of comparisons with other hospitals: comparisons in which St George's often came out as second best. From the 1870s onwards, the hospital appeared to be playing catch-up with its rivals. If the managers were not responding to the results of surveys, they were being pressured into reform by their own nurses. Few, if any, innovations seem to arise directly from the officers themselves; and the voice of Matron Coster is almost entirely absent. It is tempting to assume that her silence is an artefact of Victorian record-keeping (which silenced the female voice) rather than a failure to contribute. However, the latter may be closer to the truth. On either side of Coster's long 25-year reign were two voluble lady superintendents, whose strong views were regularly recorded in the minutes. The root of St George's difficulties in maintaining its position relative to other hospitals may lie in the timidity of Mrs Coster, at a time when those competitors had thrusting, ambitious young matrons at their helms.

How hospitals like St George's managed to attract women to work as nurses, given the competition which had arisen for female workers in other, less demanding sectors, is a continuing question. Christopher Maggs has claimed that the attraction stemmed from the development of a special status for nurses in the public's mind. He characterized initiatives such as those taken by St George's, particularly on promotion, as less important, being 'all jam tomorrow' (Maggs 1983: 20).

But this is to do nurses a disservice. If women were looking for long-term careers (which, this study suggests, must be considered likely), long-term incentives – such as promotion and regular pay awards – would be part of the attraction. Initiatives to improve conditions (particularly in terms of job content and promotion) can be indisputably linked to improvements in the hospital's ability to attract and retain a high calibre of women as nurses. Status may have been important, but so too were job satisfaction and career development.

Pen Portrait 4 Harriett Kendall – a quest for independence

Harriett Kendall (born *c.*1829) was the daughter of a blacksmith. She grew up in Spitalfields, in the shadow of the London Hospital. She probably had some elementary education, as by 1851 she was employed as a governess, perhaps for one of the silk merchants in the area.

If she had not considered nursing before, her interest may have been kindled in the late 1850s, by the publicity surrounding Nightingale and the Crimea. Around this time she joined Guy's as an assistant nurse. Guy's Nursing Department was still very much unreformed. Matron Loag had been there since 1845, as had many of her head nurses. Harriett was trained by these loyal but conservative servants of the hospital.

She stayed at Guy's for four years. Her next post points to an emerging career plan. Instead of joining another hospital, she entered one of the new nursing institutions which supplied nurses to private homes. It was a risky move: work was not guaranteed. But private nursing offered opportunities, most notably a rare degree of independence. It gave nurses a chance to hone and refine their skills and to take responsibility.

In April 1870, Harriett joined St George's. She was quickly promoted to head nurse, with responsibility for several nurses and probationers. Her job was to be the doctors' eyes and ears, taking instructions, relaying them to her team, and reporting back. If anything went wrong, Harriett shouldered the blame. She was sometimes found wanting and received two formal reprimands. Despite this, she prospered: in 1874 she was promoted to Night Superintendent, the second most important nursing post at St George's, after the Matron. She had sole responsibility for the hospital (patients and staff) at night. Should an emergency arise, it was Harriett who decided to wake the resident medical officer; not an easy decision with the prospect of a grumpy doctor roused from sleep unnecessarily. However, such disadvantages were outweighed by a significant increase in salary and invaluable management experience.

Harriett's career planning paid off. In 1876, she was made Superintendent of a Torquay-based nursing institution. Her resignation was noted with much regret, but for Harriett the thought of being in control of her own institution must have proved too strong a lure. A move to Torquay enabled her to escape grime-encrusted London for the more salubrious surroundings of the 'English Riviera'. Many of her clients would be wealthy visitors, rather than the poor who inhabited the wards of St George's.

Harriett held this post for at least 15 years. On retirement she moved back to London to care for her sister's widower. She died in 1902, aged 74, from 'decay of nature' and heart disease.

Harriett's case illustrates how a single Victorian woman could carve out an independent position in a patriarchal society. Despite her unpromising start in life, and lack of a husband, she rose to a position of respectability and great responsibility.

5 The development of nursing as a career

Few historians have studied the careers of ordinary Victorian nurses. The lives of nurse leaders have been well documented, but the experience of the anonymous majority remains largely overlooked. Christopher Maggs attempted to remedy this in studying four provincial hospitals, but was thwarted by a lack of surviving data. At one hospital, he found that, between 1881 and 1914, over 50 per cent of probationers left at the end of their training, but he could not determine what happened to them afterwards. A number left for health reasons and a relatively low number left for marriage. The high drop-out before the end of training, he assigned to poor selection criteria (Maggs 1980).

Monica Baly's examination of the early years of the Nightingale School found, on the contrary, that a 'surprising number' left to be married (1987). The data may not be comparable; Baly's nurses worked in the earliest years of nursing reform, while Maggs' data covers a period when those reforms had arguably become embedded. Women's attitudes to work and (to a lesser extent) to marriage had evolved in the interim, as discussed in Chapter 1, possibly explaining the different findings.

In Baly's dataset, 72 of 148 entries provided reasons why nurses left within their four-year contract. In addition to those who left to get married (21 per cent), 18 per cent were dismissed for insobriety and 14 per cent left through ill health. A further 26 per cent were dismissed for disobedience, misconduct or unsuitability. Only 14 of the original 148 continued in nursing beyond the four years, although this could reflect loss of contact with the women, rather than definite departure from the profession (Baly 1987).

St Thomas' policy of placing trainees in provincial hospitals, after one year's training, was a key element of Nightingale's stratgey to shape the nursing world (Abel-Smith 1960). Several became superintendents of provincial hospitals, a fact used by Nightingale's modern supporters to demonstrate her impact on Victorian nursing, but the success of this strategy has been queried, in light of the apparently large number of failed trainees (Baly 1987).

Maggs' and Baly's work constitute the entire discussion of Victorian women's careers in nursing, and this chapter will address this important gap. It will investigate the careers of St George's Hospital nurses, following their fate on leaving their *alma mater*.

Baly's surprise at the number of women who left to be married was not shared by late Victorian nursing commentators. The apparent inevitability of marriage was used as an argument against investment in nurse training. The following quote from a hospital secretary illustrates this common belief: 'Oh well!... [being dismissed would not] matter so much for her. Presumably she would give up her profession when she married and so the certificate would not be essential' (*NR*, 1 June 1895: 387). The assumption that the nurse would marry soon after completing her training, and that – once married – she would surrender all aspirations to work is a reflection of society at the time.[1]

The idea that women entered nursing merely to fill time before marriage gained strength, as its popularity among single middle-class women grew. Nursing reforms were targeted at this group; and in this, reformers were almost too successful. By 1900, nurse training schools were oversubscribed and in danger of transforming into finishing schools for young socialites.

The *Nursing Record* and *The Hospital* regularly berated the many educated young women attracted to the profession for the wrong reasons. They were described as 'naïve [recruits] who now besiege the hospitals to secure situations as probationers ... from a home of comparative ease where their hardest day's physical labour is a morning spent in light housework followed by an afternoon's lawn tennis' (*H/NM*, 9 March 1889: lxxxix). Motives of escape from home-life were ascribed to them, 'to get cured of a love affair, [or] to obtain a husband – for we all know, "love drives many in and many out of a hospital"'. Matrons were urged to differentiate between such flippant applicants and those 'who really have to earn their living' (*H/NM*, 23 March 1889: c).

Sister Grace, a regular correspondent in *The Hospital*, complained of the growing number of young middle-class women who saw nursing as an escape:

> [They have] a great deal of time on their hands ... [and] dissatisfied with their lot in life, find it dull, narrow, and uninteresting, and think they discern a picturesque opening as hospital nurses. They have read novels where the nurses ... glide from bed to bed, smoothing pillows, moistening hot brows with eau de cologne, and performing other light and elegant duties. ... The end of these charming creatures is always matrimony [with one of] ... a host of enamoured House Surgeons who hang on their smiles.
>
> (*H/NM*, 4 January 1896)

Catherine Judd traces the origins of this romanticized image of nursing to the aftermath of the Crimean War, when the 'heroic nurse' construct was formed. This figure went into battle against disease, impurity and immorality, combining religious piety and feminine innocence in a heady mix. But, if the 'heroic and angelic nurse' was intended to eradicate sexual imagery associated with the 'old style' nurse, the stratagem failed. The new nurse, in her supposedly untouchable and unattainable state, served merely to enhance the fantasy (Judd 1998: 32).

Arguably, it was this very mixture of saintliness and wickedness which appealed to the bored young women of the early 1890s, who hoped nursing would animate their lives. Large numbers saw it as an opportunity to escape the *ennui* of the drawing room. Nursing offered freedom from the family and opened up the possibility of adventure (Prochaska 1980). This romanticized view – originally constructed to attract young middle-class women – was now blamed for floods of unsuitable women applying to the profession. Nurse leaders turned to the press to demystify the work.[2]

An article in *The Lady*, in 1889, discussed the 'current overcrowding of the profession' which left 'nearly every large family [numbering amongst its members] a trained nurse' (*The Lady*, 25 April 1889: 417). The writer categorized probationers into seven 'styles', many of whom did not stay the course. The three worst were:

> The Noisy Pro ... noisy and untidy ... found her home too dull and thinks it must be awfully jolly to work for the doctor and see operations...
>
> The Sentimental Pro ... gushes to everyone about everything, [but] the realities of hospital life either curb this sentimentality ... or she gives up...
>
> The Flighty Pro ... to whom any man is attractive, and who fancies none can resist her ... generally ends in a foolish marriage ... she can hardly be regarded as a would-be nurse; a will-be wife is a truer title.
>
> (*The Lady*, 25 April 1889: 417)

Most did not survive their probationary period, but left unqualified – disheartened, disillusioned or to be married. They found the work hard and unpleasant, the patients ungrateful and often abusive, the doctors (and even their own colleagues) unimpressed by their efforts and sacrifices. Their initial self-image of bedside angel swiftly changed to that of drudge. A disappointed 'Paying Probationer' wrote to *The Hospital*, summing up the disillusionment: she had spent most of her time cleaning, washing and 'doing fireplaces'. When she left she knew 'how to do housework', but was thoroughly indignant at being 'so unfairly treated and roughly used' (*H/NM*, 7 July 1888: lvi).

Nurses as husband-seekers?

Choosing nursing for the wrong reasons was a class isssue. The 'types' described above almost certainly had not entered nursing out of economic necessity: escape, self-sacrifice and husband-hunting were clearly the prime motivations. To the last group it offered particular inducements. Unlike other occupations for respectable women – where strict segregation of the sexes was maintained – nursing involved regular contact with male colleagues, often from similar social backgrounds.[3] Finding a future husband was a realistic goal.

But, it is hardly surprising that nursing failed to live up to its romantic ideal. Once a woman joined a hospital, the job was revealed in its true nature: it was hard manual work, and the probationer was at the bottom of an extensive and strictly observed hierarchy. Additionally, their superiors – both in the nursing and medical staff – could come from lower social classes, rendering relationships potentially awkward (Summers 2000).

The image of nursing in novels and the popular press ensured that it continued to be associated with romance, despite hospitals' best efforts to discourage this. Engagements between nurses and doctors interfered with hospital discipline, distracted the nurses, and – if taken to their natural conclusion – resulted in the loss of nursing staff. According to one matron 'the doctors always chose her best nurses', a view which chimed with the belief that good nurses made good wives (*NR*, 25 May 1895: 364).[4] Dr Steele, Superintendent at Guy's, lamented how the best nurses were lost to marriage, and regretted that their names were subsequently removed from the Nurse Register. This was not the case for married lady doctors, who were permitted to remain on the register of medical practitioners (*The Hospital*, 17 December 1887). Dr Steele's views were unusual for the time; women were expected to relinquish their jobs on marriage.

The Hospital Secretary, quoted above, expounded further on hospital engagements:

> A nurse is certainly apt to lessen the discipline of her ward and relax some of her efforts, when she has love making in her head [and] the object of her affections would ... be liable to come in at odd moments.
>
> (*NR*, 1 June 1895: 387)

The same never appears to have been said of doctors, reflecting society's view that women (unlike men) were completely in thrall to their emotions (Davidoff 1983; Rose 1992).

Strict rules policing contact between hospital doctors and nurses may have helped reduce engagements between staff. At St George's, before the 1880s, rules governing nurses' behaviour made no specific mention of relationships with doctors (SGHCON/1 1873). But in 1883, a rule was introduced banning male visitors from nurses' rooms without permission, and banning medical students from the rooms of head nurses (SGHCON/1, 8 January 1883). Similar rules were introduced at the Hospital for Sick Children at Great Ormond Street (HSC), in 1897, banning all male visitors without Matron's permission (GOS/5/2/49 1897).

In 1884, the St George's rule on fraternization was further strengthened as nurses were banned from the medical school, and in 1898, unofficial communication between probationers and medical officers was banned (SGHCON/1, 10 March 1884; SGHCON/2, 10 March 1898).

Opportunities for nurses and doctors to interact had always existed, so why were such prohibitions only introduced in the 1880s? The increasing numbers of young women from 'better' social backgrounds may explain this new outward show of propriety. Throughout the 1880s, as discussed in Chapter 2, the quality of St George's nurse recruits improved, and in order to maintain high-calibre candidates, the hospital had to reassure the outside world (especially parents of prospective nurses) of the institution's propriety.

One 'Mother's' letter to the *Nursing Record* highlights the importance of a hospital being beyond reproach, and the visibility of nurses, as its public face:

> On Sunday afternoon, my ideals were shattered ... I saw a young woman in the full uniform of a well-known London hospital – smoking a cigarette ... reclining in the stern seat of a boat ... bonnet-less ... laughing loudly and in concert with two young men in boating flannels. I have decided that my daughter shall not become a nurse.
>
> (*NR*, 30 June 1894: 432)[5]

Such an image jeopardized public support, on which hospitals were financially dependent, and also threatened future recruitment. The good opinion of parents was essential for an institution hoping to recruit young middle-class women. If such women were to be permitted to leave the family home to enter the public sphere, their protection from scandal must be assured (Cominos 1980).

Other institutions where young women lived and worked faced similar challenges. An art student wrote to the *Nursing Record* that her professor had berated his students on the subject of marriage, stating, 'my school is intended for the production of artists and not for the training of wives'. Romantic entanglement was punished by dismissal – for the woman only. The writer found this rule incomprehensible, wondering why a wife and mother could not also be a fine artist (*NR*, 25 May 1895: 371).

Hospitals were in a unique situation, compared with other employers of respectable young women: their nurses had to work closely with members of the opposite sex. As Martha Vicinus argues, nursing involved 'complex problems of gender, class and status' (1985: 87). It was impossible to segregate female nurses from male officers or male patients; and it was equally impossible to ensure that they came into contact only with members of their own class. The image of hospitals, in Victorian society, was a confused one, mixing the highest form of philanthropy with an ideology which conflated disease, poverty, dirt, corruption and sin as five faces of the same phenomenon. Managers had to tread a fine balance to reassure parents of institutional respectability. But the effort was worthwhile: the arrival of middle-class women resulted in characteristics inherent in them (order, purity and morality) being transferred to the host institution (Bashford 1998).

Any hint of scandal threatened this carefully constructed image of respectability and propriety. It was, perhaps, to protect this image rather than to curb romance, that St George's introduced the new regulations regarding fraternization when it did.

How closely did stories of widespread husband-seeking among nurses reflect reality? Arguably, the problem was manufactured in the press. Magazines, newspapers and even *The Hospital*, ran hospital romances, and the public appetite for such material was great.[6] Catherine Wood condemned a romance in *The Hospital*, claiming it gave a 'false idea of the discipline and arrangements of hospital life', and '[lowered] the whole tone of moral uprightness in the workers of these institutions' (*H/NM*, 25 December 1886: 218). Her letter stimulated a lengthy correspondence. Those who agreed with Miss Wood (including Louisa Twining) cancelled their subscriptions, but Henry Burdett defended the story as innocent recreation.[7]

> [Nurses] enter upon it with the same objects as they enter any more obviously secular callings – viz for the purpose of earning a livelihood at a congenial occupation ... they no more think of barring themselves from marriage by becoming a nurse than by becoming a telegraph clerk, a secretary or a lady doctor.
>
> (*H/NM*, 1 January 1887: 236)[8]

However, *The Hospital* frequently published scathing indictments of husband seekers, and such attacks may have been an example of the didactic, cautionary literature common in the late Victorian era, designed to deflect unsuitable young women from joining the profession. Lynne Vallone has discussed the role of this type of material for girls. Cautionary tales, conduct manuals and novels with a message existed to 'tell the story of the bad girl' as a warning to those who would share her fate (Vallone 1995). Perhaps the nursing journals were using a similar device to warn off inappropriate nurse candidates. *The Hospital* and the *Nursing Record* feature husband-seeking so often as to leave the impression that marriage among hospital staff was rife, but was this true? The rest of this chapter will investigate the role of marriage and its significance compared to other reasons for departures from the Nursing Department of St George's Hospital.

Leaving St George's

By the end of the century, St George's had developed a nursing career structure which aimed to retain the best nurses for as long as possible. The system arose out of a crisis in nurse retention in the late 1860s and early 1870s.[9] In response to the crisis, an annual nursing report was instigated with detailed analysis of movements within the Nursing Department, listing the number of nurses hired by grade, promotions, resignations and dismissals (SGHCON/1, 5 July 1875). Figure 5.1 illustrates the nurse retention problems.[10] It shows the number of nurses who left each year expressed as a percentage of the nursing workforce, analysed by the main reasons for leaving: resignation, ill health or dismissal.[11] The low attrition rate pre-1870 may be attributed to incomplete surviving records. However, the gradual rise in leavers during the mid- to late 1860s mirrors a rising concern regarding the instability of the Nursing Department, recorded in the Minute Books.

From 1868 to 1888, resignation was the most frequently cited reason for leaving, although in the 1870s the problems of discipline (already discussed in previous chapters) are reflected in the high levels of dismissal.

Staff turnover in the 1860s and 1870s was most acute among assistant nurses. In 1876, one third of night nurses left during the year; but over half of the assistant nurses left in the same period (SGHWB/41, 25 April 1877). The high turnover in assistant and night nurses caused particular concern, as they were expected to fill vacancies among head nurses (SGHWB/28, 13 April 1853). The new probationer scheme, introduced in

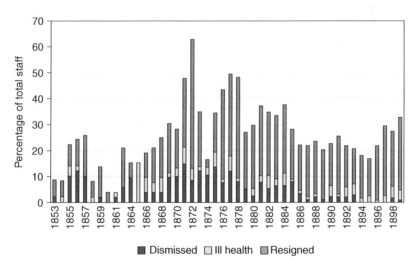

Figure 5.1 Leavers as a percentage of total St George's nursing staff, 1853–99 (sources: St George's Hospital Nurses' Database, 1840–1900).

1868, was supposed to create a pool of trained assistant nurses, from which head nurse vacancies could be filled. By moulding these trainees to the hospital's standards, it was hoped to curtail turnover and introduce stability to the Nursing Department. The initial scheme failed. The review of leavers carried out in 1875 showed that only half of the 56 probationers admitted since 1868 became assistant nurses; assistant nurses continued to be recruited from outside, as did head nurses (SGHCON/1, 5 July 1875). The main reason for leaving was resignation, suggesting either the hospital or the work was failing to meet expectations.

Exploding the marriage myth

Earlier in this chapter it was suggested that, contrary to contemporary accounts, in fact few women had marriage in mind when they enrolled as probationers. It has already been suggested (in Chapter 2) that the minimum age for recruits was set at 25 to avoid loss of women to marriage, it being assumed that most women who wished to marry were, by then, either wives or fiancées (Maggs 1983). If true, then it seems unlikely that hospitals would be affected by large numbers of nurses leaving to be married.

Between 1876 and 1893, St George's Committee of Nursing recorded the number of nurses lost to marriage in its annual reports. The numbers were very small. The highest incidence (in 1878) accounted for only 7.8 per cent of nursing staff, the figure normally being below 3 per cent – or two nurses a year of 20 leavers in total. This explodes the myth that marriage was a significant drain on nursing departments (at St George's at least) and supports Christopher Maggs' findings (1980). These data suggest that the image of nursing as a stop-gap between school and marriage, did not accurately reflect reality; and that it might have been created by various pressure groups to promote political objectives.[12]

Marriage was often most closely linked to paying probationers in the nursing press. It was alleged that these women (who generally signed up for short three- to six-month schemes) never intended to make a career out of nursing, but behaved like the 'Flighty Pro' encountered earlier. Perhaps the whole profession became tainted by a 'marriage myth', based on the behaviour of this small, unrepresentative but high-profile group of nurses. Letters from career nurses accused paying probationers and lady nurses of flirting with the idea of nursing, at the expense of their own livelihoods.

One anonymous contributor to the *The Hospital* wrote:

> Is it just, that ladies with large incomes ... who because of the restlessness of the age or some disappointment, should rush into the nursing world and take the bread from those less-favoured gentlewomen who have no resource but to work for their living?
>
> (*H/NM*, 8 June 1889)

Writing ten years later (indicating that this was an enduring problem), another complained about lady nurses taking employment from those who genuinely needed it. She noted that this was not exclusive to nursing, having seen a letter in the daily press complaining of 'lady journalists' who took work away from trained female journalists who needed the work (*H/NM*, 4 March 1899).

The evidence from St George's, which supports the argument that marriage rates among nurses were not excessively high, should be viewed in the light of the absence of paying probationers there, if the two phenomena were indeed linked.

If nurse-marriage was not a major concern for St George's, the Weekly Board's growing worry was those who left for new jobs or who were dismissed. These two categories accounted for over 65 per cent of all departures. Using the database created for the study, it has been possible to produce a detailed analysis of leavers. Figure 5.1 shows the number of dismissals declining in the late 1870s, while resignations remained high throughout the 1870s and early 1880s. They fell off in the period between 1886 and 1895, only to rise steeply again in the last four years of the century.[13]

The dismissed

Dismissals reached a peak in 1871, when 15 per cent of nurses left for this reason. The process of dismissal was formal as Nurse Sarah Newton's case illustrates. She had been suspended by the Matron for insolence towards herself and the Night Superintendent, after being reprimanded for rule-breaking. Summoned to appear before the Committee of Nursing to defend her behaviour, she failed to keep her appointment and was dismissed (SGHCON/1, 29 January 1872). Her dismissal probably resulted from her insolence and failure to attend the hearing, rather than the original infringement. Her case illustrates the limits of Matron's authority, she could suspend a nurse from duty but could not dismiss her.

The dismissals are broken down into four categories: conduct, disobedience, unsuitable and insobriety. Dismissal for breaches in conduct included 'quarrelling', 'improper conduct', 'absence without leave', 'misbehaviour', 'unclean in habit', 'cruelty' and 'theft'.[14] Disobedience included 'insubordination' and 'broke rules'. Dismissals in the unsuitable category reflected recruitment errors, nurses being described as 'unsatisfactory', 'not strong enough', 'not suited' or 'inefficient'. The last major category, insobriety, is self-explanatory. A fifth category, 'other', included women for whom no reason was given for their dismissal and those made redundant in Nursing Department reorganizations (see Figure 5.2).

The hospital's policy of training its own nurses in order to improve behaviour appeared to work. From the 1880s, there was a steep decline in those dismissed for bad conduct, insobriety or disobedience. By the end of

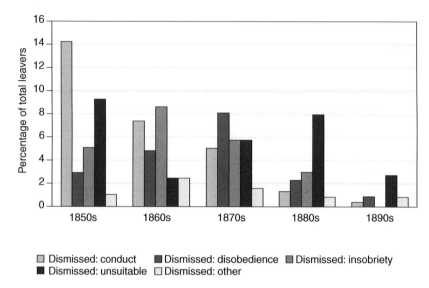

Figure 5.2 Reasons for dismissal from St George's as a percentage of total number of leavers (sources: St George's Hospital Weekly Board Minutes, the Committee of Nursing's Annual Reports and the Nurse Registers).

the century the very few dismissals stemmed from inappropriate recruitment, that is, women who proved to be unsuitable for nursing.

However, prior to the 1880s, indiscipline and unacceptable behaviour were rife. Poor conduct covered a wide range of behaviour which upset the smooth running of the hospital, or had the potential to damage its reputation. Quarrelling or theft disrupted discipline within the wards and caused potential danger to patients. Cruelty to patients and poor hygiene could result in real harm; while improper conduct (that is, inappropriate relationships between the nurses and male members of staff or patients) had potentially disastrous consequences for the hospital's public image.

Quarrelling between head nurses and their assistants was rife. In 1874, the Committee of Nursing received a letter from patients complaining about the head nurse of Oxford Ward (SGHCON/1, 2 March 1874). The investigation revealed that Assistant Nurse Hobley had instigated the letter, presumably in retaliation for some slight against her by the head nurse. She was called before the committee and reprimanded (SGHCON/1, 20 March 1874). A few months later, Hobley was dismissed after staying out all night. The combination of the two incidents, so close together, was probably more disobedience than the committee could tolerate (SGHNR/2 Hobley).

Absence without leave was one of the most common infringements. In a hospital which was always chronically short-staffed, illegal absence undermined duty rosters and put patients' welfare at risk. The lengths to which the hospital went to address this problem indicate the extensive control it exerted over its nurses.

When a woman signed up as a nurse at St George's, she handed control over her life (both inside the hospital and outside) to the Matron and management. Although free time increased throughout the century (as the benefits of rest and fresh air were appreciated), access to time off was very controlled. Signing in and out were mandatory, even for two-hour breaks, and permission was required for longer absences. From 1871, a book was kept at the porter's lodge, 'in which should be recorded the time a nurse leaves and returns to the hospital, and this book to be laid before the Committee of Nursing whenever it meets' (SGHWB/36, 6 December 1871). Nurses who infringed their leave entitlement were confronted with this evidence. Whether other members of staff had their movements monitored to this extent is unclear. The records do not suggest that doctors, medical students or even female domestic staff were subject to similar scrutiny.[15]

Such surveillance was not unique to hospitals. Women's colleges enforced regulations to control and protect their female students. Newnham, in the centre of Cambridge, insisted that its students were chaperoned about the town (Tamboukou 2000).[16] Girton, however, situated in the countryside (and therefore without such intense social surveillance) permitted its students more freedom. The college doors were still locked at 10 p.m. every night, and any woman caught returning later faced expulsion. Teacher-training colleges exercised similar control over students, again threatening tardy returnees with dismissal (Tamboukou 2000). Discipline was there to protect reputations, both of the institution and its members, but hospitals had an additional need: while reputation was important, control of nurses' movements was essential to ensure the smooth running of the wards.

Live-in female shopworkers also faced scrutiny, and the doors to their hostels were closed at a specific hour (Whitaker 1973). An 1880 manual on suitable work for women emphasized the benefits of shop work: evenings were entirely at workers' own disposal, and they were 'allowed' to go away at the weekends, if their employer knew their whereabouts (Grogan 1880). As with nurses, there were probably two facets to these controls on shopworkers. Employers regarded themselves *in loco parentis* and the reputation of their employees, and (by association) their stores, had to be upheld. At the same time, shopworkers' hours were extremely long and late nights were hardly conducive to good time-keeping and alert sales assistants. As in the hospitals, shop-owners needed to ensure the efficient running of their establishments.

St George's nurses' explanations for their late return sometimes stretched the bounds of credibility. Night Nurse Coppens claimed to have assisted at an unexpected birth, when she had been visiting two servant friends in the house of a lady. She produced a letter to corroborate her story, but a lengthy investigation by Harriet Coster finally revealed the letter to be a fake, and the lady non-existent (SGHCON/1, 7 May 1872). Having been caught out in a lie, Coppens asked for permission to resign (SGHCON/1, 10 June 1872). Dismissal was an undesirable outcome for all concerned, and the option to resign was often offered as an alternative to dismissal. From the nurse's point of view dismissal was disastrous – the end of her career; without a good reference her ability to find alternative employment was severely limited. Too many dismissals also reflected badly on the hospital, suggesting poor discipline and a lack of moral strength in its workforce. Dependant on public contributions, voluntary hospitals could not afford such stains on their character. The practice of allowing nurses to resign rather than be dismissed may indicate that dismissal levels were under-reported, with a proportion of resignations 'at own desire' representing nurses who jumped before they were pushed.

This flexibility could only stretch so far. For the persistent offender, or for a grave offence, dismissal was the only outcome. Night Nurse Ruby (who had been at the hospital for nearly two years) pushed the limits of the managers' tolerance at Christmas 1872. She requested leave to be absent for the whole of Christmas Eve night. Her request was denied, but she went anyway, returning at noon the following day. She was dismissed immediately. Ruby had committed this offence before, and her repeat offending probably accounted for the harsh punishment (SGHCON/1, 20 January 1873).

Alongside breaches of conduct, disobedience was also a key reason for dismissal, especially in the 1870s. Discipline was at the heart of nursing, and disobedience was simply not tolerated. It usually took the form of acting against orders or flouting established rules and regulations. One example illustrates how the wrath of the hospital could fall immediately upon a nurse who chose to ignore instructions.

In May 1870, a notorious murderer, Walter Miller, was admitted to the hospital. He had tried to kill himself as he was being arrested and his subsequent trial was covered in national newspapers (*Pall Mall Gazette*, 13 May 1870). The presence of such a celebrity in the hospital must have caused quite a stir. The managers ordered his head nurse to forbid anyone, including other nurses, to see him. Overcome by curiosity, Louisa Gamble, head nurse of another ward, demanded to be allowed in. When her colleague tried to prevent her, she reportedly said, 'she did not care, others had done so and she would do so too' (SGHNR/1, Gamble). Gamble was reported to the Committee of Nursing and dismissed immediately, despite having served in the hospital for over five years. Her deliberate flouting of a very specific instruction, and its challenge to the authority of the hospital managers, could not be tolerated.

A less frequent cause for dismissal was improper conduct. This usually involved inappropriate relationships with either a male member of staff or a patient. In 1891, Ward Nurse Ada Wilcockson was suspended for 'improper behaviour in the wards with male attendant Deacon'. The Committee of Nursing reported that, 'unseemly conduct has recently existed between Nurse Wilcockson and the attendant Deacon, especially on or about the 12th instant, when she allowed him to take her up in his arms' (SGHWB/54, 19 October 1892).

Both nurse and male attendant were dismissed immediately.[17] This type of behaviour could not be tolerated in the hospital, where outward propriety was essential. Wilcockson and Deacon placed the hospital managers in a very awkward position, providing visible evidence that they had failed in their duty to protect her reputation. It is interesting to note that both Wilcockson and Deacon were dismissed, in contrast to the outcome of relationships between nurses and doctors, where only the nurse could expect this censure.[18] Presumably for Deacon, both his class and his lowly position in the hospital hierarchy counted against him.

The worst offence in the category of improper conduct was for a nurse to become pregnant. There was no more public display of rule-breaking than a pregnant nurse. Assistant Nurse Olivia Chapman, a young widow, was reported to have been 'confined on the night of 28 December 1870, and was warded in Burton'. Chapman had concealed her condition well, her head nurse stating that she had no idea of 'Nurse Chapman's state' (SGHCON/1, 9 January 1871). Her entry in the Nurse Register noted, '[The] lady disgraced herself' and she was discharged immediately (SGHNR/1 Chapman). A nurse of the same name and age has been traced in 1871, working at the Tonbridge Union Workhouse, so it appears that she was able to find a new position, despite the disgrace (SGHNDB). No trace of her child has been found. In another case, Night Nurse Kerry was dismissed (in 1875) after being discovered to be pregnant. The Register recorded that she was 'enceinte' (SGHNR/2 Kerry).[19] Both Chapman and Kelly were widows and had clearly conceived out of wedlock. In Chapman's case, given she had been at the hospital for 15 months there was no doubt this had occurred while she was in the hospital's employ (SGHNR/1 Chapman).

Pregnancy among single women was the ultimate Victorian taboo. It carried total loss of respectability for the woman, whose physical condition was testament to the fact that she had breached the protective barriers thrown around her.[20] Chapman and Kelly were lost causes, but it was not just their reputations at stake. The reputation of the hospital was also endangered, and it had to take the necessary steps to repair the damage.

Cases of improper conduct were rare. More significant was the caricature of 'old' Victorian nursing: the inebriated nurse. As Figure 5.2 illustrates, dismissal as a result of intoxication was a rumbling problem at St George's up to the early 1880s. The variety of terms used to describe drunkenness among the nurses (inebriation, intoxication, drunkenness, intemperance and insobriety) illustrates its importance in the Victorian psyche. Some nurses returned from leave in a state of intoxication, presenting themselves as unfit for work, while others were discovered to be drunk (or drinking) on duty. Although the image of the drunken nurse was common, at St George's it was a low level (if persistent) problem: during the period of study only 30 nurses in total were dismissed for being drunk. However, when it did occur, the managers took steps. Night Nurse Anne King, who had been at the hospital for only a few months, returned drunk from unsanctioned leave – a double infringement – and was dismissed immediately (SGHWB/33, 9 August 1865). Her daughter, who had been a nurse at St George's for nearly two years, felt compelled to resign, 'in consequence of her mother's misconduct' (SGHWB/33, 30 August 1865). The daughter had not transgressed, but her mother's shame rendered it impossible for her to remain.

Although the hospital would not tolerate drunkenness, it provided its nurses with a beer ration as part of the daily diet. During the 1880s and 1890s, head nurses repeatedly requested 'beer money' instead – as was the practice at most large London hospitals – but this was always refused (SGHCON/1, 9 July 1877; SGHCON/2, 11 February 1895). The hospital may have been attempting to control nurses' intake, by keeping their disposable income to a minimum; or, mirroring state intervention in alcohol consumption, it could be seen as a strategy to encourage nurses to drink beer rather than gin.[21] Beer was considered beneficial for those engaged in heavy work. It was also thought to protect against infections such as typhus, scarlet fever and diphtheria (Rafferty 1996: 15).

Moderation was the key and inebriation amongst nurses was not to be tolerated. Tough punishment was meted out to offenders as a warning to all. From 1887, inebriated nurses were examined by the Resident Medical Officer (RMO), who reported to the Committee of Nursing (14 March 1887). By the late 1880s, insobriety amongst the nurses was diminishing and disappeared completely during the following decade. Did this result from the hospital's tough alcohol policies or the changing demographic, which saw more middle-class nurses in residence; or did it reflect shifting societal attitudes towards drinking and drunkenness? F.M.L. Thompson has suggested that changing attitudes towards alcohol, favouring temperance but not absolute prohibition, emerged as the century progressed (1988: chapter 8). It seems likely that a general change in drinking habits was responsible for the disappearance of this problem among St George's nurses, rather than any action of the hospital.

Nurses and ill health

Popular myth decreed that nursing ruined a woman's health, but, on average, only 2.6 per cent of St George's nursing staff left through breakdown of health in any year, and the death rate in service was even lower. This study has identified 33 nurses' deaths between 1850 and 1900, equivalent to just over one nurse every two years or a death rate of 1.14

per cent.[22] *The Times*, in 1869, claimed that the annual death rate for nurses at St Bartholomew's (Bart's) was 3 per cent, compared with a 'normal death rate' for females age 33, of 1 per cent (*The Times*, 27 October 1869: 9). The investigation of the London Hospital reported four deaths a year, equivalent to a death rate of 1.8 per cent (*Pall Mall Gazette*, 25 September 1890). Death among St George's nurses was, therefore, similar to the death rate for females in a comparable age group in the general population, and lower than that at either the London or Bart's. Given their poor accommodation and lack of leisure time, this is somewhat unexpected.

Public interest in the state of nurses' health was sparked by press coverage of the 1889 House of Lords' Report into the Sweating Industries, and further fuelled by the sensational revelations regarding nursing at the London a year later (HoLSC/MH 1890). Nurses, and their parents, deluged the newspapers with letters claiming their health had been ruined by nursing. One father wrote that his daughter's well-being had been destroyed by hours of cleaning and scrubbing during her training as a children's nurse (*Daily News*, 5 January 1889: 6). *The Queen* argued that overwork and poor diet led to an inevitable breakdown of nurses' health (19 July 1890).

A nurse from Bart's, on the other hand, argued that, for fit women, the work was not damaging to health. Those who complained, she wrote, were those who had not given serious consideration to its nature before signing up (*Daily News*, 14 January 1889). Another pointed out that, unlike typists and clerks, should she fall sick a nurse was given the very best medical treatment, free of charge (*H/NM*, 7 December 1895).

Letters such as these, however, did not change the general public perception that nursing was bad for the health. The *Pall Mall Gazette* summed up its view:

> In hospital everyone is cared for except the nurse, who is considered simply as a machine wound up by imaginative enthusiasm, set going by the opposition of friends, and expected to work night and day until a spring breaks and life is useless … almost always on their feet, breathing the exhalations from diseased humanity … subjected to many insults, obliged to hear oaths and coarse language – to work, work, work until at last their short life of usefulness is over.
>
> (*Pall Mall Gazette*, 3 April 1889: 3)[23]

How different from the lives lived by many young middle-class women at the end of the century. Typical days consisted of a social round of visits and intellectually unchallenging pastimes such as letter-writing and needlework, while evenings were filled with trips to the theatre, parties and more visiting (Dyhouse 1981: 43). In such circumstances, they were prone to become vacuous, superficial or 'mysteriously ill' (Vicinus 1985: 14).

In contrast, those single women who – freed from family responsibilities after the death of parents or other dependants – chose to travel abroad to 'wild places ... for reasons of frail health ... found themselves, once abroad miraculously cured of their dyspepsia, depression and *ennui*' (Perkin 1993: 159). Escaping the stultifying family environment could improve the health of the sickliest socialite, and, it was argued that nursing could have a similar effect. A probationer writing to *The Standard* claimed that, far from being damaging to health, nursing was much healthier than being at home. She described a friend, who, being a 'very delicate girl', found nursing work 'very hard and very trying'. But once at home, the constant social round and late hours left her more exhausted than when she had been working. The writer concluded that 'the regular hard work of hospital life is less trying than the irregular hard work of many girls who live at home' (*Standard*, 9 March 1889: 2).

Ethel Fenwick, while believing nurses were not inherently in danger, advocated more attention be paid, lest the work should damage their health. In an article entitled 'The Overstrain of Nurses', she claimed that in one large training school (almost certainly the London), one-fifth of probationers left within a few months, because of 'loss of health'. She urged hospital administrators to tackle the problem, which stemmed from the psychological stresses of close contact with the sick and dying, a lack of access to fresh air and exercise, and a poor and irregular diet (Fenwick 1889).

Fenwick advocated more free time for nurses and improved accommodation and diet, but such remedies required funding and nursing departments appeared to be last in line when money was handed out (*Standard*, 8 March 1889). At St George's, as discussed in the previous chapter, leave for assistant nurses was repeatedly delayed in the face of opposition from their senior colleagues (SGHCON/1, 9 July 1877). When monthly leave was finally introduced, one head nurse resigned, claiming that this left her impossibly short-staffed (SGHCON/1, 9 July 1877 and 22 August 1877).

The Hospital, in its role as mouthpiece for hospital administrators, showed scant sympathy on the issue. It claimed that probationers 'who broke down' brought it on themselves. Some women had underlying health problems. Others, having entered nursing for the wrong reasons, were made miserable by the work and their psychological state produced physical debility, leaving them susceptible to infection and deteriorating health (*H/NM*, 20 August 1892). At St George's, in the 1890s, nearly 9 per cent of probationers left early, 14 through ill health and three because they were 'not strong enough'.[24] Half of these left within the first six months, supporting Ethel Fenwick's observation that probationers were at greatest risk in the early stages.[25]

At St George's, nurses' ill health was not serious enough to cause many resignations, but there was a constant level of sickness which disrupted the hospital's routine. Illness was a major cause of lost working days and for an understaffed hospital (as St George's was regularly described), the loss of nurses from the wards must have disrupted patient care.

The RMO's annual report to the Committee of Nursing included a narrative on nurses' health and statistics on the incidence of sickness. The standard measure used was the 'Mean Daily No. Sick', calculated from the total number of days lost to sickness in the year, divided by 365, providing an average number of nurses absent on any given day. Figure 5.3 plots this for the 17 years it was reported to the Weekly Board. Up to 1890, the 'Mean Daily No. Sick' was generally under four, but in the early 1890s, it rose steeply, peaking at 7.29 in 1893. This huge rise was explained entirely by annual influenza epidemics between 1889 and 1894, which hit the Nursing Department hard.

The influenza pandemic of 1889–94 (known in Western Europe as Russian flu) caused over 150,000 deaths in Britain. In London, the worst affected UK region, roughly a third of inhabitants were affected, with doctors and nurses being among the first to succumb. High levels of initial absenteeism disrupted commerce, further exacerbated by the 'thousands of convalescents ... [left] weak and depressed, in debt and unfit for ... work' (Smith 1995). Workers in the public sector suffered prticularly: over 20 per cent of Post Office Savings staff and one third of telegraph operators were afflicted; 21 per cent of workers in London branches of the London and Westminster Bank, and 20 per cent of booking clerks in the London and Northwest Railway Company (Smith 1995). At St George's, at its height, 37 nurses out of a staff of 88 were affected. Many suffered relapses and ill health all year, possibly due to returning to work too soon,

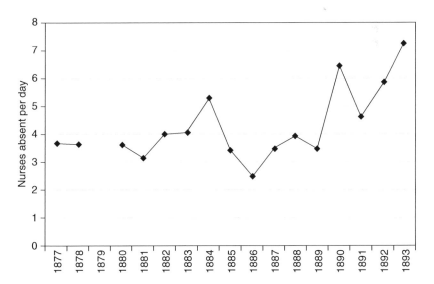

Figure 5.3 Daily sick rate among St George's nurses (source: St George's Committee of Nursing Annual Report on Nurses Health 1877–93).

but also reflecting the long-term effects of influenza (SGHWB/53, 1 April 1891).

Extraordinary cases also produced dramatic effects on the hospital's statistics on nurse health. The peak seen in 1884–5 was explained by the long sickness of a few nurses, rather than deteriorating health in general (SGHWB/49, 22 April 1885). The fall in sickness observed in 1886–7 was particularly noted, the RMO's report stating that '[the rate] of under 3 per cent of daily sickness among [nurses] appears ... to speak well for their general management and treatment, and thanks of the Governors are especially due to the Superintendent of Nurses' (SGHWB/50, 6 April 1887). It is not clear what actions, if any, had brought about this improvement, but it was short-lived, reversing the following year.

Obviously concerned by the high level of background sickness, the committee attempted to obtain similar statistics for other hospitals, but it was reported that 'none seem to be available' (SGHWB/47, 4 April 1883). The matron of the Middlesex did confirm that the daily sick rate at her hospital seemed to be 'much the same as at St George's (SGHWB/47, 4 April 1883).

Given the public outcry about nurses' health, did nurses suffer more than other women workers? A common measure of sickness in a community is prevalence, in this case, measured as the number of sick days per nurse per year.[26] If sickness prevalence is calculated for St George's nurses, the statistics can be compared with other sources.

Using this measure, sickness among St George's nurses was found to be more prevalent than in the working population as a whole, according to data from James Riley's work on a friendly society's medical records.[27] According to Riley, sickness prevalence among male members of the society rose from 9.0 sick days per member year in 1872 to approximately 12.5 in 1900. Unfortunately, the equivalent data for female workers was not available, as the society did not admit women until 1892, and between 1892 and 1898 their numbers were statistically insignificant. Data from 1898 to 1915 indicates that female sickness rates were lower than their male counterparts, ranging from 6.75 to a peak of just over 9.0 in 1915 (Riley 1997: 167).[28] The data for St George's suggest much higher sickness rates, averaging 19.4 sick days per nurse per year, for the period 1877 to 1893. While Riley's population and time period are not directly comparable, his study appears to provide some evidence that sickness was more prevalent among St George's nurses than among other working populations.

So, although nurses' health was not sufficiently impaired to cause them to leave, their poor general health affected the efficient running of the hospital. Many of their most common afflictions were chronic and prone to recur. They included rheumatism, bronchitis, gastric problems and sore throats. Infectious diseases, such as scarlet fever, diphtheria, typhoid, measles and mumps also featured, but not as often as might be expected in a hospital environment. This could indicate that nurses had developed a natural immunity. Despite the existence of the Metropolitan Asylums Board (MAB)'s specialist fever hospitals, St George's still admitted cases of infectious fevers, particularly diphtheria (which were excluded from the MAB hospitals until the late 1890s), and its nurses came into daily contact with them (Ayers 1971).

Most surprising is the complete absence from medical reports of tuberculosis (TB), one of the major causes of mortality in the general population throughout the period (Hardy 1994). Why was this? The disease may have been misdiagnosed as bronchitis, which was a frequent cause of sickness among the nurses, or possibly, cases were deliberately hidden by the RMO. TB was a heavily stigmatized disease and the doctors may have wanted to protect the nurses, and the hospital, from the shame attached to it (Hardy 1994). Debbie Palmer, in her study of nurses' health in several institutions, has also noted this phenomenon (Palmer, personal communication, August 2009). Riley found much lower incidence of the disease than he expected, and suggests a medical reason for its absence. As TB is a chronic condition (which often progresses at a very slow rate), he postulates that it is feasible that workers with TB became incapacitated long before a positive diagnosis could be made (Riley 1997: 194–5).[29] The true incidence of TB at St George's may be hidden among the nurses who left under the general category of breakdown in health. (See Pen Portrait 2: Eliza Ockenden, p. 73, for the story of a nurse who died from the disease.).

Another unexpected finding is the comparatively low incidence of accidents or injury in the RMO's report on nurses' health. They may have been recorded separately, in records which have not survived, but even so one would expect to see a summary of time lost due to injuries. Most surgical cases in the RMO's report appeared to be the result of accidents – finger abscesses (probably the result of infected cuts) and acid burns predominate – but this detail was only recorded in three reports (SGHWB/45, 13 April 1881; SGHWB/46, 19 April 1892; SGHWB/48, 26 March 1894). Lifting injuries were completely absent, although conditions associated with repetitive pressure on joints, such as rheumatism, occur frequently.[30] Perhaps lifting injuries were too trivial to be included? Records of nurses being issued with support stockings and trusses suggest they occurred but were not included in the statistics, possibly because they were endemic (SGHWB/30, 10 March 1858).

Initiatives taken by managers to improve working conditions appeared to have no impact on nurses' sickness levels, but a different picture, one of declining levels of ill-health, might emerge if the effects of the influenza epidemics of the early 1890s could be removed from the analysis. The data do not allow this, but Figure 5.3 does appear to show a gradual decline in absence through ill health before those epidemics occurred.

Nurses who resigned

The Committee of Nursing's Annual Reports analysed the reasons for nurses' resignations. This source is more comprehensive than the Nurse Registers or Minute Books and provides insight into almost every resignation between 1876 and 1893. As with dismissals, terms used in the original records to describe the reasons behind resignations, have been grouped together to enable analysis, under the following headings: 'new job', 'unhappy', 'end of training', 'personal reasons', 'retired' and 'no reason'.

The single most important reason for resignation was to take a new job, although, from 1888 to 1891 'end of training' was frequently cited (see Figure 5.4). This latter reason coincides with the introduction, in 1885, of the three-year contract for probationers (SGHWB/49, 22 April 1885). By this time, as already discussed, the hospital trained more nurses than it needed, and those leaving at the end of training probably had no choice, there being insufficient staff nurse posts for all the newly qualified probationers. By 1892, leaving for a new job again became the most frequent reason for leaving, as 'end of training' disappeared. The change may merely reflect a change in recording practice. In the early years of the three-year scheme, the hospital may have used 'end of training' to recognize the success of the new training programme. However, once its existence became less of a novelty, there was less need to emphasize it.

Dissatisfaction was a major cause of resignations, particularly in the 1870s. Recorded in the Committee of Nursing minutes as 'unhappy', it took many forms, including discontent with the conditions under which

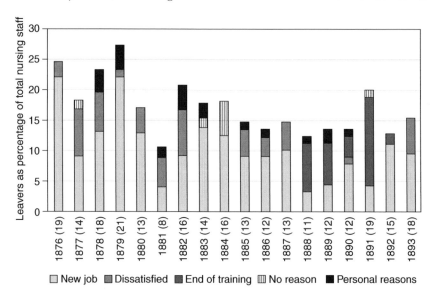

Figure 5.4 Reasons for resignation from St George's (source: St George's Committee of Nursing Annual Reports, 1876–93).

nurses worked.[31] The increasing attention paid to the comfort of nurses, from the 1880s onwards, seems to be reflected in a general improvement in nurses' contentment, and a decline in resignations for this reason.

Nurses were unafraid to express their feelings. Food was 'not of good quality & not properly cooked', said one on her resignation; another complained that she 'had to go into the open air to count dirty linen' and also had to clean her own room (SHGCON/1, 28 November 1870; SGHNR/1, Collins). The latter, Thomasina Collins, joined as head nurse, having trained at St Thomas'. During her time there, she may have formed a view of what constituted acceptable working conditions for a head nurse and found St George's wanting.

There also seems to be some correlation between resignation and reprimands. Nurse Caroline Bellamy had been publicly accused by the house surgeon of disobeying an order. Believing herself to be innocent, and humiliated by the public rebuke, she resigned. The Committee of Nursing exonerated her, and offered to reinstate her, but she remained firm. It was noted in the minutes that Nurse Bellamy 'left with no stain on her character' (SGHSCON/1, 9 April 1872; SGHWB/36, 12 April 1872).[32]

In other cases, nurses resigned to pre-empt a worse fate, to safeguard her character and all-important testimonials. A campaign against Head Nurse West, who was known to '[have] a very bad temper and is most arbitrary with her nurses', ended in her resignation in 1880. Complaints against West came from patients and nurses on her ward; and a night nurse reported her drunk on duty. She was cleared of all charges except that of bad temper. Despite this, West handed in her notice before a more serious fate could befall her. That the committee accepted her resignation 'on account of her previous good service' suggests she had narrowly avoided dismissal (SGHCON/1, 18 August 1880).

In separate incidents, nurses Ann Farrow and Elizabeth Clarke resigned, shortly after being reprimanded for reporting a patient's condition directly to a doctor, rather than their head nurse. They had flouted the strict hierarchy in the hospital. Although the reprimands were not linked to the women's resignations in the committee minutes, the juxtaposition of both events suggests a causal relationship. Perhaps admonishment was the final straw for two women already dissatisfied with their lot (SGHNR/2 Farrow; SGHNR/2 Clarke).

By resigning, such nurses left with their characters intact, retaining good references. The hospital managers appreciated the importance of these references, and used the threat of withholding them to good effect. Ruth Phillips, a ward nurse who joined the hospital in July 1881, was warned that, if she left before completing 12 months' service, her testimonial would be withheld: she wisely delayed handing in her resignation until September 1882 (SGHNR/3, Ruth Phillips).

The focus on good testimonials indicates that, for many St George's nurses, their work (and earning a living) was important. They would do what was necessary to ensure their continued employment elsewhere, if their future did not lie at this hospital. For the hospital, it was often preferable to accept a nurse's resignation than to risk a scandal, or have doubts cast on discipline.

St George's nurses were far from the docile and submissive creatures of nursing mythology, as these examples indicate. They were set on careers, and prepared to stand up for themselves. Several of those dissatisfied with conditions at St George's have been found in subsequent censuses working in other nursing jobs, including Thomasina Collins, who by 1871, had been appointed Superintendent of Nurses at the Greenwich Hospital for Seamen (SGHNDB).

A smaller group of resignations relate to personal reasons; often the result of nurses returning home to care for a sick relative or widowed parent. Although society was gradually more accepting of working middle-class women, the traditional duties of a daughter and sister continued to make a strong claim on a single woman's freedom. In domestic tragedy or crisis, it was to single women that the burden of care fell, as they were expected to return to the traditional role as 'the family's surrogate mother' (Vicinus 1985: 10).[33] Nurse Ann Jinks resigned from St George's in 1871 to nurse her sick mother. She was permitted to return four months later; but when her mother fell ill again in 1877, she left immediately (without the required notice) and was told this time not to come back (SGHNR/2 Jinks). Widow Susan Crandle, on the other hand, left because 'she was anxious to live at home and take care of her [two young sons]' (SGHWB/34, 22 May 1867). Prior to joining the hospital, Crandle had worked as a seamstress. By 1871, having left St George's, she resumed this work and was living with her family. The higher wages in nursing could not, in the end, compete with the claims of her children.[34]

When Nurse Josephine Stanley's children caught scarlet fever, in 1870, she asked for leave to look after them. The hospital insisted that she pay for a substitute to cover her absence: she could not afford the cost and resigned. As she had not given the statutory notice, the Matron stopped three weeks' wages. This particularly harsh treatment appeared to be punishment for lying about the size of her family: on joining she had admitted to one child, when in fact she had two. Despite this, the Matron still provided a good reference, stating she was 'good medical nurse' (SGHNR/1 Stanley).[35] This enabled her to find work the following year as a private nurse (SGHNDB).

New jobs

The main reason for leaving throughout the period was to obtain a new job. The Committee of Nursing's Annual Reports give an indication of the type of job nurses left for, and additional sources allow a more detailed picture of nurses' careers to be created. In some cases, the registers provide information not just on the initial job after leaving, but also on subsequent positions. Nurses would return to their *alma mater* for references years after leaving, and kept the Matron up to date with their progress.[36]

Increasingly detailed records of nurses' careers, kept by the *alma mater*, became the norm as the debate on nurse registration intensified, reflecting the growing need for nurses to have proof of 'good' training, and a record of their experience. The pro-registrationist lobby placed a central system of nurse training and certification at its heart, proposals which were vehemently opposed by large metropolitan hospitals. They wished to retain control over their own nurse training, and contended that only they could comment on a nurse's efficiency. As a member of this group, St George's had to demonstrate it was capable of producing and maintaining reliable records, or risk providing fuel to the pro-registrationist argument. This would explain the appearance, from the ealy 1890s, of such details in the St George's registers. The hospital encouraged ex-nurses to remain in contact to enable their careers to be monitored.

Increasingly, nurses left the hospital for other jobs in nursing (see Figure 5.5). By the end of the century, of all those traced, less than 10 per cent were outside the profession.

In the mid-nineteenth century occupations open to respectable women were few. Employment was largely restricted to domestic servants, governesses and lady companions; but by the end of the century the situation had changed. The *Nursing Record* published a series of articles in late 1889 entitled 'Women and their Work', featuring an array of potential

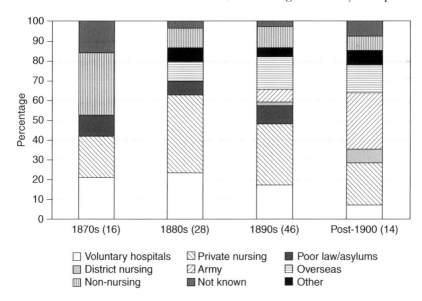

Figure 5.5 Subsequent nursing roles of nurses who left St George's (source: St George's Hospital Weekly Board Minutes, 1850–99; St George's Hospital Committee of Nursing Minutes, 1868–99; St George's Hospital Nurse Registers, 1870–99).

occupations for women: lady clerk, schoolmistress, lady shop assistant, boarding-house keeper, dressmaker, Christmas card painter, journalist, post office clerk, waitress, and even lady dentists.[37]

Between 1861 and 1901, women clerks in the census grew from 279 to nearly 58,000. They worked in commercial enterprises, including law firms and insurance offices. Over the same period the number employed in the civil service (mainly in the Post Office, as clerks or telegraph and telephone operators) rose from 2,000 to just over 25,000. In comparison, nurse numbers grew at a much slower rate, from around 25,000 up to 64,000, although nursing was still one of the largest single groups (Holcombe 1973).[38] On the surface, many occupations appeared more attractive than nursing. They offered more freedom, shorter hours and in some cases higher wages; although once a nurse's living expenses were taken into account the wage differential was greatly reduced. The basic salary for a Post Office clerk in 1897 was £65, while female commercial clerks could expect to earn £52 a year (Holcombe 1973; Anderson 1988; Davin 2005). The best manufacturing jobs could earn female operatives nearly £50, while teachers in the new public schools could earn £100 a year (Anderson 1988; Jordan 1999). A staff nurse's wage of £20 to £25 a year does not look very attractive in comparison, but if a value of £50, for board and lodging, is added to the nurse's salary, her wage rises to £70 to £75, and is more comparable with other jobs.[39]

Teaching is perhaps most easily comparable to nursing as a profession for single women, and a study of teachers in teacher training colleges has revealed several parallels, in terms of career development, with St George's nurses (Robinson 2000).

Like many nurses at St George's, these women (employed by local school boards to train elementary school teachers) came predominantly from lower social class backgrounds, and their chosen career offered an opportunity for improvement. Training was long; they remained unmarried throughout their working lives and were prepared to move around the country to further their careers. Robinson has described them as 'often highly ambitious, career minded and committed to their personal education and professional development' (Robinson 2000: 101).

Shop work was also a growing sector, which some similarities to nursing: many workers lived in, the hours were long and the wages low. In *How Women May Earn a Living* (a self-help book published in 1880), shop work was described in glowing terms. The shop girls interviewed professed themselves 'happy' and felt much better off than 'if they were governesses'. Their accommodation was described as 'spacious' and 'airey', and their food as 'plentiful and good'. Like nurses, young shop women were often employed on an apprentice basis. At Howell & James, which employed lady shop assistants, women were required to sign a three-year contract and pay a premium of £40 (Grogan 1880: 92).

Grogan's description of occupations needs to be treated with scepticism. She described nursing accommodation thus: 'liberal board and comfortable bedrooms … always provided', a description which bears little resemblance to nurse accommodation at St George's (Grogan 1880: 72). Whitaker, on the other hand, has described shopworkers' conditions as cramped and overcrowded; with poor food, little time to take it, an overwhelming number of rules, and very long working days, mostly spent standing. With wages of £15 to £40 per annum, by the end of the century, their conditions of work were comparable in many respects to that of nurses at St George's (Whitaker 1973).

It is significant that, with an increasing pool of occupations to choose from, so many St George's nurses chose to stay in nursing after the 1870s. Few, if any, left to work as clerks or shopworkers. Age could be a factor in that. Telegraphy schools, for instance, preferred girls aged 14–18, while the civil service employed women aged 18 and above (Davin 2005). With a lower age limit of 25 for new nurses at St George's, and an obligatory three-year contract, a nurse was likely to be at least 28 on leaving the hospital, possibly too old to move into a new field. By the end of the century, employers generally came to favour young impressionable women and ex-nurses were probably far from ideal candidates. Too old to enter a new occupation as a trainee, lacking the skills for a higher position, ex-nurses were barred from these new occupations. But more importantly, how attractive would such a move be to a newly qualified nurse? If a nurse left with good references and a first class certificate, it made sense to use those skills in their future occupation.

One of the few non-nursing jobs which appealed was as an independent trader, especially to older women close to retirement. Some of the older nurses from St George's have been discovered as confectioners or laundry owners – businesses which they may have set up using savings or their hospital pension. Jane Burchett, a head nurse at St George's, chose to move into retail on retirement. On her resignation in 1855, on the grounds of ill health, she asked the Board to 'take into consideration my past service of 12 years 4 months, and tender me a little assistance to enable me to open a shop for the sale of trifling articles'. The minutes recorded that having received good character references from the Matron, Apothecary and Steward she was awarded the sum of £10 (SGHWB/29, 7 March 1855).

Ann Moseley (see Pen Portrait 3, p. 108, for full details) also turned to shopkeeping in her retirement. Nursing had enabled her to rise from very humble beginnings, to improve her social status to that of small business owner.

A career in nursing

The majority of St George's nurses elected to remain in the profession. As Figure 5.5 indicates, by the 1880s, of all nurses traced, nearly 90 per cent were found in nursing jobs. A trained nurse had a wide range of nursing jobs to choose from. She could move into Poor Law nursing in asylums, workhouse infirmaries and fever hospitals; become a private or district nurse; transfer to a specialist hospital, such as a children's hospital, or undergo further training to become a midwife. Some found posts as matrons of convalescent homes, often in salubrious surroundings.[40] Later in the century, nurses chose to join the colonial or army nursing services, using their training to travel overseas.

In the 1880s and 1890s, private nursing accounted for between 30 and 40 per cent of nurses who left for new jobs. It offered better wages, freedom from institutional life, the choice of when to work and the opportunity to be one's own boss. For nurses with children, it offered flexibility, and the chance to return to the family home. There were disadvantages. There were no paid holidays, no free health care nor paid sick leave, and although wages could be higher, there were many hidden costs, not least having to pay for board and lodging when not working. Independent nursing also carried dangers. Working within private homes, a nurse was frequently exposed to intimate, but unchaperoned, contact with the opposite sex, in a way few other female domestic workers were and in an environment very different from that in hospitals. Philippa Hicks, Superintendent of the Nurses' Cooperation, said of private nurses:

> Few outsiders are aware of the tremendous temptations and perils in the life of a private nurse ... the nurse is young, often good-looking, her patient may be a man ... [and] there are critical moments when danger is very close.
>
> (*St James Gazette.* 29 November 1892: 12)[41]

A private nurse had to be constantly on her guard.

There were two options for private nurses: she could work on her own, developing a network of medical contacts and clients; or, she could join one of the nursing institutes.[42] These offered the safer option, acting as placement agencies for nurses and providing a base when they were not working. Some provided benefits such as holiday and sick pay. The downside was the level of wages: the practice of charging high rates to clients, but paying low wages, generated a great deal of resentment amongst their employees.[43]

In 1890, a group of nurses, tired of the perceived exploitation of their labour, founded the Nurses' Cooperation (*H/NM*, 10 May 1890). Backed by Henry Burdett, its first Lady Superintendent was Philippa Hicks, who had been persuaded out of early retirement from the HSC to take on the role.[44] The Cooperation found placements for its members who, in return, paid 7.5 per cent of their earnings to cover running costs. At the end of the year, any profits were shared. Earnings averaged 2 guineas a week. At this rate, a woman could earn the equivalent of a hospital nurse's annual salary in just three months (*H/NM*, 5 September 1891). The Cooperation became very popular, and by the end of 1891 it was turning nurses away.[45] It opened a residential club in 1892, where nurses could obtain meals and meet friends; and also provided overnight accommodation for nurses who needed 'an occasional bed' between appointments, or a permanent address for correspondence (*H/NM*, 19 March 1892). The success of the Cooperation shows that nurses could take their destiny into their own hands.[46]

By 1895, with the exception of the Cooperation, nursing institutions were finding it hard to fill vacancies despite offering good salaries and comfortable living quarters. The difficulties were blamed on a culture among nurses to be 'independent':

> The almost universal spirit of restlessness and discontent with anything but what people ... call 'an independent position' is rapidly degenerating the nurses of today. ... Every trained nurse wishes either to be in a post of authority ... or if private nursing be her special line, then she must be 'independent'.
>
> (*H/NM*, 7 September 1895: clx)

Many nurses found the freedom and independence of such employment attractive. Despite it being precarious, with no sick or holiday pay, the rewards were potentially great. An independent private nurse wrote that she earned £140 in one year, equivalent to £90 in a hospital (*NR*, 3 February 1894).[47] This is substantially higher than the wages of a staff nurse (£35–£45), or even a sister (£50–£65).

Private nursing also offered the opportunity to work in upper-class homes. This could confer on lower-class women a rise in social status, by association. For nurses from higher social classes, who worked through economic necessity, private nursing could offer them a route back into a society which they previously inhabited. Mrs Jordan, a character in Henry James' novella, *In The Cage*, illustrates this strategy well. A clergyman's widow, left penniless, she set herself up as a personal florist to high society. By visiting their houses regularly she explained, 'one seems to live again with one's own people' (James 2001: 326). Later, trying to persuade her friend to join her in the business, she promised to 'send you to all the bachelors', offering the young girl the hope of entering (or re-entering) society through marriage (James 2001: 330). Private nursing, with its affluent middle- and upper-class clients, had the potential to generate similar opportunities (SGHWB/49, 22 April 1885).[48]

By the 1890s, however, many of the nurses at St George's were looking further afield (see Figure 5.5). They appear to have been both an ambitious and an adventurous group. As the Committee of Nursing commented in 1885, it must be expected that large numbers of 'young nurses [will leave each year] given the great demand there now is both at home and abroad for educated nurses, and the prevalent love of change' (SGHWB/49, 22 April 1885).

By the end of the century, nurses from St George's were dispersed across the world. Several travelled to South America to work in hospitals in Rio de Janeiro and Buenos Aires.[49] In 1893, St George's nurse Sarah

Clayton went to Rio to take up work in the Strangers' Hospital. She had been a domestic servant before entering nurse training. For Sarah, nursing must have opened up horizons beyond her in other circumstances. Unfortunately, the Brazilian adventure had an unhappy ending. Tropical illness hit the hospital and two nurses died, one of whom was Sarah. Her matron, in reporting the deaths, described Sarah as a 'most valued and efficient Nurse' (*NR*, 3 November 1893: 295).

Frances Burtwell also ventured to Brazil. She had trained for six years, at Sydenham Children's Hospital and then at St George's. At the time of her appointment to the Strangers' Hospital, in 1899, she had been a sister at St George's for 18 months. She left for Rio in a party of three other nurses (*NR*, 2 September 1899: 189).

Other popular destinations for St George's nurses included India, in particular the Bombay Plague Hospital, and the Rangoon Municipal Hospital in Burma. Isabella Leitch trained at St George's and completed one year as a staff nurse before taking up the post of sister at Rangoon, in 1898. By 1902, she had been appointed Matron (*NR*, 11 January 1902). A less happy outcome awaited Florence Morgan, who left St George's in 1897, after three years' training, to become a sister at the Plague Hospital in Bombay. She was promoted to acting Lady Superintendent a short time later, but died of the plague in February 1898 (*NR*, 19 February 1898). The *Nursing Record* carried many announcements of the deaths of nurses working in hospitals overseas, usually from the tropical diseases they had gone to nurse. Death from plague in India and Burma, and yellow fever in Rio, were not uncommon. Despite these dangers, women continued to take up posts abroad, their search for adventure and promotion overcoming any reservations. By the 1890s, over 20 per cent of St George's leavers went to nurse overseas: many under the auspices of the Army Nursing Reserve, set up in 1894 by the Royal British Nursing Association (and supported by Princess Christian) to provide a reserve of nurses to serve in the army during times of war. Others went to the Colonial Nursing Association, established in 1896 (Summers 1988; Rafferty and Solano 2007).

There are fewer references to nurses travelling to the USA, Canada or the Antipodes. In 1886, Annie Sharp asked the Weekly Board for permission to apply for the post of 'Superintendent [of Nursing] to the Hospital of the University of Pennsylvania'. The Board provided her with a glowing testimonial, which commended her for,

> The energy, zeal & efficiency with which she has performed her duties ... in the service of this Institution ... Miss Sharp has given entire satisfaction to this Board, & while they would regret losing her services ... they feel assured that if chosen for [this] important post ... she will ... prove a valuable acquisition to the Pennsylvania Hospital staff.
>
> (SGHWB/49, 31 March 1886)

Annie Sharp did not get the job: there were 79 applicants, the successful candidate being Charlotte Hugo, 'a Nightingale school graduate' (Stephenson 1940; G. Farr, private communication, 18 April 2006). Annie's subsequent fate remains unknown, but the fact that she felt able to apply for such an important job indicates the quality and ambition of the women who nursed at St George's in this period.

By the turn of the century district nursing was also a popular option. This trend mirrors the rise of the Queen's Nursing Institute (QNI), a highly organized nationwide group of district nursing organizations. The QNI presented itself as a professional institution which maintained close scrutiny of its members and a 'roll' or register which listed their qualifications and experience. Nurses who did not maintain the required standards were removed from the roll (Sweet and Dougal 2008).

As Figure 5.5 indicates, most St George's nurses left the voluntary sector to continue their careers, but a small number gained further experience within it, prior to applying for more senior posts. They travelled around Britain, as they had been prepared initially to travel to London to train (as discussed in Chapter 2). Most, however, stayed within southern England, and those who moved outside London moved to smaller towns rather than the large conurbations. One reason for this could be the presence of existing nurse training schools. By the end of the century, Birmingham, Manchester, Liverpool and Leeds all had large teaching hospitals with well-established schools of nursing. It is likely that vacant positions, both in these hospitals and also in the myriad of cottage hospitals in their immediate vicinity, were filled primarily from this local reservoir of trained nurses. Nurses from St George's were also competing with nurses from other London training schools, and, although it was well respected, St George's did not appear to have the same reputation as St Thomas' or Bart's, as Annie Sharp's experience proved.

Robinson's study of teacher-trainers has found a similar pattern of movement within the profession. One third of female teachers in teacher centres moved 'around the circuit', and the majority moved over substantial distances, although she does not discuss any regional bias in these movements. Women were more likely than their male colleagues to change jobs more than once, some moving three or four times in the course of their career.[50] She also found that moves were not always in search of promotion, and that some teachers moved back and forth between the centres and the schools. This mirrors the nurses' habits of moving between private and hospital nursing, and indicates that both groups of women pursued their craft in a variety of settings (Robinson 2000).[51]

As with Robinson's teachers, most St George's nurses who moved to another hospital did not move for promotion but to take up similar roles. Some went to specialist hospitals, such as Moorfields Ophthalmic Hospital, or Stockwell Fever Hospital; others into the state system. Ellen Mary

Parham left St George's in 1898 to become a private nurse, but by 1901 she had moved into the Poor Law system, working at an Essex workhouse infirmary. Subsequently, she worked at two workhouses in Kent, before her last entry in St George's Register (in 1905) when she was at the 'Benefit Nursing Asylum' in Woking (SGHNR/6 Parnham).

Alice Raynes had promotion in her sights as she moved around the system. Trained at St George's, she had reached the position of sister when she left the hospital to go to a fever hospital, 'to gain experience of fever nursing'. She returned to St George's in 1897 as Matron's Assistant, and having held that post for a year, was able to obtain the post of Matron at Banstead Fever Hospital in 1898 (SGHNR/6 Raynes).[52]

St George's nurses were clearly prepared to move to further their career. The relatively few openings for promotion within the hospital forced this. Of 90 nurses whose careers outside the hospital have been traced, over 15 per cent eventually reached the position of matron. Most went to provincial hospitals: Leonora Biscoe became Matron at Chelmsford Hospital, while Susan Carvosso was elected Matron at Salisbury Infirmary and then moved to Derby Royal Infirmary. One of the few exceptions was Mary Roberts, who trained at St George's and held the post of head nurse there for four years before being appointed Matron at Queen's Hospital, Birmingham (SGHNDB).

Isabella Brown was another exception. Her case illustrates several important aspects of building a career in nursing: a preference by teaching hospitals to employ their own nurses in positions of authority; the importance of networks; and the effect of networks on mobility. Her nursing career began with three years' training at Pendlebury Children's Hospital in Manchester. She moved to London to take a staff job at King's, to gain adult nursing experience, and in 1896 she was appointed sister at the HSC, under Florence Smedley. In 1898, she followed her old matron to St George's, to become one of the first externally recruited sisters. She remained at St George's for nine years, after which she returned to King's as Assistant Matron (SGHNR/4 Brown, I.; GOS/5/2/1). The networks she had built up during her early years in nursing were obviously instrumental in determining the course of her later career.

Despite the success of this small group, the majority of St George's nurses remained as staff nurses, meeting the demand for hospital nurses caused by the explosion in bed numbers during the latter part of the century. They tended to remain in London and the south of England, but worked at a wide variety of hospitals, including workhouses, district infirmaries and asylums. Few moved to other large metropolitan hospitals to take up positions, possibly reflecting the fact that, like St George's, these institutions preferred to employ nurses they had trained themselves.

Conclusion

By the end of the century nursing had become diverse, with branches and specialisms which offered careers to women. Studying the career development of nurses who trained at a large hospital like St George's can help understand the importance of this occupation. Unlike other employment open to women in the second half of the nineteenth century, where the inevitability of marriage was viewed positively by employers, marriage was not seen as inevitable for nurses. One private nurse, explaining this, wrote '[that women] who have put their hand to this plough find a fascination about their work which doesn't diminish and makes it hard to give up' (*H/NM*, 4 August 1888). Instead they trained and worked with the intention of developing nursing into a life-long career to support themselves. Some looked for adventure, being drawn to work abroad; others were ambitious, hoping to become matrons of their own hospitals. A significant number were attracted by private nursing and the quite unusual level of independence that it offered to single women (*H/NM*, 4 August 1888).

That women increasingly viewed nursing as a career, rather than just another job, is demonstrated by the lack of movement from nursing into other occupations. Before the 1880s, women frequently moved between nursing and domestic service, but with the introduction of nurse training schemes, and the increasingly technical nature of the work, nursing and domestic service began to diverge. Trainee nurses made significant investment in acquiring specialist skills, and they were not prepared to squander that. As nursing grew in respectability, it conferred improved social status on women from working-class backgrounds, and offered all (of whatever class) an opportunity to define themselves by their role in society, rather than as wives, mothers or daughters.

St George's nurses appeared to take their careers seriously and responded well to changes, staying longer, behaving better and embracing education. The number of dismissals – high in the middle decades of the century – became insignificant by its close. Problems with discipline had all but disappeared, and by the 1890s the main reason for the few dismissals was unsuitability for the job. Ill health was a constant problem, but not to the extent that the publicity surrounding nursing and women's health suggested. The death rate among St George's nurses did not differ significantly from the death rate of similarly aged women in the general population.

By the end of the century, most nurses who left the hospital did so to take up other nursing jobs and, as the hospital trained more nurses than it needed, this posed no problem. Improvements in education, accommodation and conditions of service meant it was able to attract and retain highly qualified and competent nurses. At the same time, a possibly unexpected result of these improvements was the creation of a group of ambitious women who were adventurous and independent, often looking for new experiences of the world. These were women on a quest for indepence, quite removed from the docile, saintly nurse of myth.

Pen Portrait 5 Henrietta Diller and Harriet Bailey – sisters in nursing

Henrietta Diller and Harriet Bailey were typical of the nurses who worked at St George's before the introduction of nurse training schemes. Both came to nursing after the deaths of their husbands. The unusual aspect of their story is that they were sisters.

They grew up in Bermondsey, daughters of a leather worker. Henrietta was the elder, born *c.*1820, while Harriet (or Hannah as she was also known) was some ten years younger. Nothing is known of Harriet's earlier life, but as a young woman Henrietta had worked in several occupations. In 1841, she was teaching, probably at one of the charity schools which provided education for London's poor: possibly the same school she attended as girl. It was common for schools to recruit their best pupils as teachers. By 1851, Henrietta had abandoned teaching for sewing, and two years later she married Frederick Diller, who, like her father, worked in leather. They had a daughter who died at an early age, and a son, who survived to adulthood. The marriage lasted barely three years. Diller died of tuberculosis in 1856, and a familiar tale emerges of a young widow left to fend for herself and her child. Henrietta decided to enter nursing, and by 1861 she was at Bart's.

A similar fate befell her sister. Harriet also married and had a child, before widowhood forced her into nursing. She also joined Bart's, and by 1859 she had moved to St George's as an assistant nurse. It is unclear who took the first step into nursing – but one must have influenced the other. In 1864, Harriet was promoted to head nurse and she was joined by Henrietta, initially as a night nurse. Henrietta was promoted to head nurse a year later.

The two women are among the signatories on a letter sent by head nurses to the Committee of Nursing in 1869, complaining about the Matron's demand for a pass-key to their bedrooms. They were also present throughout the turmoil of the early 1870s, when several experienced head nurses left under a cloud. But they survived. In 1870, Henrietta asked if her sister (recently moved to the hospital's new convalescent home at Wimbledon) could return to the main hospital to fill a vacant head nurse post. The request was granted. Of the two, Harriet seems to have been the more highly regarded. In 1879, her name was put forward by the hospital to become a St Katherine's nurse – a great honour bestowed by the Queen herself. It carried an honorarium of £50 a year for three years.

The two sisters continued to work together until Henrietta's retirement in 1881. Harriet retired several years later. Both received pensions.

The importance of nursing to working-class women, as a means of support when their worlds collapsed, can be seen in the stories of Henrietta and Harriet. So too can the influence of family. Nursing provided both with a means of financial security, and in Harriet's case, in particular, public recognition of the skills she had acquired.

6 A quest for independence

The origins of modern nursing cannot be understood by focusing exclusively on the development of the occupation as a profession or on studies of the handful of women who battled for its recognition. Such an approach, while undoubtedly having a place in nursing history, produces institutionalized accounts based on a public image constructed by its leaders, thus subsuming the reality of what happened on the wards. This approach cannot address questions about the lives of nurses who worked in the voluntary hospitals, and who burgeoned in number in the second half of the nineteenth century. Questions concerning the origins of women who became nurses, their motives for choosing that occupation, the experience of being nurses in the second half of the nineteenth century, and how their lives unfolded as a result, remain unaddressed by the traditional historiography. Yet such questions, if they were to be asked, could shed light on the nature of nursing and would also contribute to an understanding of the experience of working women in Victorian Britain. Little attention has been paid to nursing by women's historians or labour historians. This may be because its development appears – on the surface – to offer no great breakthroughs, insights or paradigm shifts. Just as it might be argued that the history of the family has been overlooked, as a result of its association with the everyday and the mundane, perhaps the same fate has befallen nursing, with its close connection to domesticity. The portrayal of nurses as self-sacrificing angels has served to repel further late twentieth-century feminist historians for whom traditional religious allegiance and seeming conventionality present little attraction.

This study seeks to redress some of these omissions. It is based in the tradition of microhistory, and answers Maggs' call to study nursing from below. It further develops his use of hospital records by including data derived from census records. The prosopographical techniques employed have introduced a new methodology to the discipline. This book demonstrates that novel questions – previously considered unanswerable as a consequence of the dearth of direct evidence – can be addressed by linking information from a variety of sources. A study of nursing from below, as presented here, reveals new testimony on the lives of ordinary women;

evidence which challenges the traditional assumptions on the experience of Victorian women.

The approach is unique in several respects. It is the first to reconstruct the lives of a group of Victorian nurses, tracing them as children with their families, through adulthood and into retirement. The combination of information from archival nursing records and data extracted from decennial census records has generated unprecedented detail on a cohort of nurses in the second half of the nineteenth century. It has enabled, for the first time, the class structure and profile of a nursing department at a major Victorian voluntary hospital to be monitored over a 50-year period. The results challenge many of the traditional views of Victorian nursing.

Solidly working-class in the 1850s, by the end of the century the Nursing Department at St George's had experienced an influx of middle-class women. Despite the rhetoric of nurse leaders (suggesting a wholesale gentrification had occurred), St George's nurses continued to come from a wide range of backgrounds. The hospital accepted women into its Nursing Department based solely on their suitability for the work and treated all women the same. Significantly, it had no 'special probationer schemes', as was common at other prestigious London hospitals. By the mid-1890s, it was reportedly rejecting 600 applicants a year, but half its probationers still came from the 'labour aristocracy', suggesting that these women were being positively selected, rather than accepted through lack of more suitable alternatives. Middle-class women who joined the hospital may have been prepared to overlook its lack of special provision in return for its address in one of the most salubrious environs of London. This desirable situation may also have had a positive influence on working-class women looking to improve their station in life, and to work in one of London's more pleasant areas.

In other respects, late nineteenth-century St George's nurses conformed more closely to the 'ideal nurse'. They became younger as the century progressed, and thus recruits were more likely to be unmarried. These attributes were a function of a recruitment policy designed to reduce costs, rather than the result of an ideological belief that young, single women made better (or more malleable) nurses. As the hospital increasingly relied on probationers to nurse the wards, and filled its vacancies from this pool, the average age of members of its Nursing Department naturally fell. At the same time, the likelihood of these women being married also declined.

The introduction of the probationer scheme was associated with a desire to improve the quality of the Nursing Department, but was arguably more closely aligned to a need to address instability in the department. For the first 20 years, it served more as a fixed-term contract (preventing women from leaving) than as a method of attracting a 'better class' of woman through the provision of specialized training. The very late appearance of compulsory lectures – and even later introduction of examinations

– is testament to this. As the probationer scheme was expanded, it conferred an additional benefit on the hospital, in reducing the cost of care for increasing numbers of patients. By the end of the century, the majority of nurses on the wards were probationers, who earned considerably less than their qualified colleagues. The economic benefit of the scheme was, without doubt, one of main motivators behind its introduction to an organization constantly struggling to maintain financial equilibrium.

Analysis of nursing records has indicated that the most frequent reason for a nurse to leave the hospital was to take up a new job. Dismissal became increasingly unimportant as the perceived general behaviour of nurses improved, while loss to marriage was never the major problem described in the popular press. Equally, the level of resignations due to ill health was relatively low throughout the period, while the death rate among nurses appeared to be roughly equal to that of women of a similar age in the community at large. This is not to say that the health of nurses was unimportant. The hospital lost a large number of working days to sickness, and took several initiatives to improve the health of its nurses, including the provision of more suitable accommodation and increasing off-duty time.

It has been possible to trace the careers of some of the women who left the hospital to take up new jobs. The results indicate that they were willing to move around the country in pursuit of their next post. By the 1890s, it is clear that some saw nursing as a starting point for adventure and advancement, moving overseas to places as far afield as India, Burma, South Africa and Brazil, often to take up superintendent posts.

In the early years of this study the department was blighted by a high turnover in staff, many nurses staying for less than a year. They left expressing dissatisfaction with the work, with their colleagues or managers, or with their living conditions. The probationer scheme (backed up by other initiatives including the internal recruitment policy and provision of improved accommodation) brought stability to the department, and by the early 1890s, the hospital trained more nurses than it had vacant staff positions. The rejected, newly qualified nurses took their highly prized certificates and went in search of work within the burgeoning healthcare sector. While some were clearly seeking promotion (which had become an elusive goal within the hospital as a direct result of its success in improving staff retention) others may simply have been looking for a fresh environment in which to practise their newly acquired skills. Few women, having invested a significant amount of time in their training, left nursing for other careers. The lifecycle data indicate that those entering the hospital often brought with them experience from other sectors (such as teaching and domestic service), but, by the end of the century, were rarely found to move into these areas after leaving. Of those women who could be traced in subsequent censuses, by the end of the century only 10 per cent were found in non-nursing roles, and many of those could be said to have retired. This was a marked difference from earlier in the century, when a significant number moved into other occupations, in particular, domestic service. It is possible that these women were using nursing to improve their opportunities of obtaining more senior positions in a domestic household. The data is not robust enough to support conclusively such a contention, but it is a plausible argument that the skills acquired whilst working in an hospital might have prepared a woman to take on senior roles, such as housekeeper, in a large private house. By the end of the century, however, a move into domestic service was much less likely, suggesting that nursing was becoming a career for women, with a clearly defined structure, rather than a branch of domestic service, as it had been regarded in the 1850s and 1860s.

A further aspect of nurses' lives came to light in the course of analysing database records. Some evidence of networks between St George's nurses has begun to emerge. There are instances of families (mothers and daughters) working at the hospital, examples of women whose families were neighbours arriving at the hospital within a short period of time, and instances of contemporaries from the hospital located in later censuses at the same address. The importance of these networks warrants further study, especially in the light of the assertion, by some historians, that nurses did not form close supportive communities.

The use of St George's administrative archives alongside data from Nurse Registers has enabled the monitoring of the effect of management initiatives on nursing staff. Thus, a correlation has been demonstrated between the extensive revisions of the system of nursing (which took place during the 1870s) with instability and dissatisfaction within the department; the fragility of the relationship between a matron and her nurses has also been exposed.

The study has revealed some insights into the character of the women the hospital employed. The tendency to ill-discipline was gradually eradicated through the entrenchment of the hospital's policy to limit recruitment to probationers, and to fill all senior vacancies internally. However, this is not to assume that these women fit neatly into the Victorian image of nurses as docile, passive and submissive. There are enough examples of St George's nurses speaking out on their own behalf, to cast strong doubts on that view. They petitioned for pay rises, more time off duty and improved living conditions; preferring to present their case to the male managers personally, rather than rely on the intercession of the Matron or doctors.

Despite proudly declaring itself to be the first hospital to invite Florence Nightingale to be an honorary governor, St George's appeared to have an ambiguous and inconsistent view of her system of nursing. In 1869, it was described as possessing a 'modern' Nursing Department, having recruited a lady superintendent to manage it; but by 1897, it was regarded as 'old', with an 'old style' matron. It was one of the first to introduce a three-year probationary period, but was among the last of the major London hospitals to formalize training, with a detailed curriculum backed up by theory and practical exams. When examinations were introduced in the early 1890s, the poor performance of probationers – especially in basic procedures such as bandaging and wound dressing – revealed deep-rooted deficiencies in the Nursing Department, suggesting that progress to develop 'new nursing' was slow. Little evidence remains to assess this progress, although the doctors increasingly declared themselves happy with the standard of nursing in the hospital. However, the large number of reforms instigated by Miss Smedley (after her appointment as Matron at the end of the century) and particularly her reluctance to use internal promotion suggests a low opinion of the quality of nursing. How much of the perceived deficiency can be laid at the door of Mrs Coster, who presided over the department for half of the whole period of this study, is difficult to ascertain. Her voice is rarely heard in the minutes (unlike her very vocal successor), but there are indications that she was of the 'old school', and may not have been sympathetic to reform.

The evidence from St George's has been compared with published information regarding nursing at other London hospitals, although it should be noted that no nursing department (with the possible exception of St Thomas'), has been investigated in the same depth. One invaluable source is the Charles Booth archive, held at the London School of Economics. It contains a unique collection of interviews with leading matrons from London hospitals in the mid-1890s. Original transcripts present these influential women's views on a range of topics, from the type of women who entered the service to the policies of the hospitals for which they worked. They reveal the conflicting opinions of nurse leaders at the end of the century, and illustrate the often contradictory relationship between the public presentation of nursing and its reality.

The relationship between a hospital and its nurses has been described by many historians as being patriarchal, infantilizing the women and placing them in a subordinate role. The overall impression of the nurses at St George's, and their relationship with the hospital's male managers, is somewhat different. Although the managers did exhibit this type of behaviour, in their control of the nurses' free time, for instance, or in their response to inappropriate relationships, there is a lack of rhetoric in the archival records to suggest that the moral element of nursing (so heavily emphasized by Nightingale and her followers) was overly stressed. As Smedley's comment regarding nurses' entertainment in the late century suggests (see p. 133), they believed their nurses were mature, intelligent women, capable of taking responsibility for their own lives. Where male managers did intervene, it was the hospital's reputation, rather than the women's well-being, which was their primary concern.

In the late nineteenth-century, nurses at St George's came from an increasingly diverse background, but once within the hospital walls, they formed Christopher Maggs' melting pot, with the only hierarchy of importance being that of the Nursing Department. To middle-class women, the hospital offered a respectable occupation with training and prospects, which enabled them to support themselves and break free from the often stultifying family life which might otherwise have been their lot. To working-class women, it offered a respectable job and promotion prospects. It also presented a chance to rise up the social hierarchy of Victorian England. The classless nature of the Nursing Department at St George's seems to contradict the image portrayed in Victorian literature, suggesting that contemporary accounts were based on the rhetoric of the reform movement, rather than reality of the wards.

There is no doubt that women flooded into nursing in the last decade of the nineteenth century. Historians have argued as to the causes of this increased popularity (particularly among the middle classes) of an occupation previously characterized – or caricatured – as inhabited by old, unskilled widows. Opportunities for women had emerged in many different occupational fields as the century came to a close. They moved in large numbers into commercial offices and the civil service as clerks, telegraph operators and telephonists; into teaching, at all levels; and into the retail trade as shop assistants. Smaller numbers made inroads as doctors, dispensers and librarians (Jordan 1999: Holcombe 1973). With these seemingly more respectable (and easier) options open to women who either wanted to work, or were forced to (through their personal circumstances), why did so many choose nursing; and what can their choice tell us about the type of women who did so?

While many of the jobs listed above (outwardly at least) appear more attractive than nursing, they shared characteristics which may have made them less appealing. In the case of office work, for instance, historians of women's labour have argued that women were only accepted into commercial offices under very tightly controlled conditions. Admitted into 'women-only' departments, which undertook the company's routine and mundane clerical work, female workers were paid low wages (in comparison to their male counterparts) while access to promotion into even junior managerial roles was blocked (Anderson 1988). Unlike in nursing, employers seemed to relish the inevitability of marriage among their female employees, as illustrated by the comment from Frank Scudamore, an early proponent of female telegraphy operators in the Post Office:

> Permanently established civil servants invariably expect their remuneration to increase with their years of service. ... Women, however, will solve these difficulties for the Department by retiring for the purpose of getting married as soon as they get the chance.
>
> (quoted in Jordan 1999: 13)

This inevitable 'natural turnover' in staff helped to keep wages down and suppressed ambition. For many employers, women offered a source of low-waged workers. With expectations of promotion severely curtailed by the inevitability of marriage, they also provided a malleable staff, available to take on the routine work, freeing male colleagues to climb the career-ladder. Such jobs offered women a brief opportunity to earn some financial independence, but no long-term prospects for advancement.

It has also been argued that many opportunities which opened for women at this time occurred as a result of deskilling of previously skilled occupations. Holcombe has used this argument in her explanation of the increasing numbers of female shop assistants; and it has also been used to explain the feminization of office work (Holcombe 1973). Ellen Jordan contends that office work was deskilled long before women began to move into it, but that the second wave of deskilling (which followed the introduction of typewriters and other forms of mechanization) opened the door to women workers (Jordan 1999). The advent of typewriters and other mechanical tools might have been expected to increase the technical nature of clerical work, and therefore create an image of a skilled occupation. But in reality such skills were easy to acquire, often at school or from one of the burgeoning suppliers of evening classes. Such was the supply of commercial courses that employers were under no obligation themselves to provide training for their female employees; and with a plentiful supply of self-trained replacements, high turnover of staff did not interrupt the business and wages could be kept low (Anderson 1988).

Contrast this with nursing. Nursing offered a very different proposition to other common female occupations of late Victorian England (with the exception of teaching). Developed as an (almost) exclusively female occupation, there was no need for structures which would artificially protect the careers and prospects of existing male colleagues. Rather, as this study has illustrated, nursing offered a well-defined structure which provided not simply a traditional career progression, but opportunities to move into different branches of the work where new skills could be acquired.

The acquisition of this valuable skills-set also sets nursing apart from most other female occupations of the time. Women were beginning to break through into other forms of skilled employment, such as medicine and dispensing, but at this period their numbers were so small as to be unimportant for most women looking for career choices (Jordan 2002). Unlike office work, where skills became demeaned by easy access, nursing skills could only be acquired on the job. Consequently, hospitals were obliged to invest heavily in both time and money to train their nurses to required standards; and such investment generated a very different relationship between the employer and employee. Whereas business managers, with no investment in their female clerks, were more than happy to see employees come and go, hospitals battled constantly to prevent a similar turnover in their nursing staff, to ensure some return on their investment. The very different reaction to the 'inevitability' of marriage illustrates this well.

For hospital managers, probationer schemes represented an investment in the future, in addition to being a very useful tool for suppressing wages during the training period. As this study has shown, by the end of the century hospitals were staffed almost exclusively by lowly paid trainees, who helped to keep costs to a minimum when finances were being squeezed. However, this was not a one-sided bargain, and women who signed up for nursing were prepared to endure exploitation of their labour in return for the very important certificate which acknowledged the valuable set of skills the holders possessed. From here, the world (literally, in some cases) was their oyster, and doors opened up to promotion, overseas travel, independent private nursing or myriad other opportunities in the many different nursing sectors. This type of two-way contract between employer and employee was not in evidence in most other forms of female employment.

Jordan has argued that women (and particularly their parents) would have been attracted to nursing by the traditional Victorian family values expounded by the hospitals, which were more strongly in evidence than found in other acceptable female professions such as teaching (Jordan 1999: 144). The residential nursing school offered a chance to escape claustrophobic family life, while at the same time retaining much that was familiar. Even if the standard of accommodation was not high, and the level of surveillance was seemingly as great (if not worse) than at home, such conditions would only endure as long as the nurse remained within the hospital. This could be as short as three or four years. After that, she was free to choose a completely independent life as a private nurse, which many did. That relatively short time invested in acquiring the right to an independent long-term future might have been a calculation many women found attractive. Other residential female workers (such as shopworkers) would experience the same low standards of accommodation and high standards of scrutiny, but with no goal in sight other than marriage.

Age was another differentiating factor which held nursing apart. Whereas most employers took young women directly from school or college, nursing schools generally set a minimum age of 23 years or even older. The effect of this was to delay the decision to enter nursing until a woman was considerably more mature than those entering other occupations, and possibly had given more reflection to the choice. As a result, as found in this study (and in Christopher Maggs' work) the impact of marriage on nursing departments in the late nineteenth century appears to have been minimal. Unlike some employers discussed above, the marriage of nurses was not regarded as a benefit, to keep turnover high and wages low, but as a waste of valuable hospital resources. Ellen Jordan has argued that probationers were treated like male apprentices, employed at low wages in large numbers to bear the brunt of nursing, but discarded at the end of training, there being insufficient staff positions to satisfy the full complement of trainees. She argues that turnover due to marriage was one way the hospitals dealt with this (Jordan 1999: 142). From this study, it can be argued that Jordan's reading of the hospitals' strategy regarding probationer schemes is too simplistic. While there is no doubt that the economic argument holds true (i.e. that hospital managers saw in probationers an opportunity to staff their hospitals for relatively low cost), this was not the sole benefit such schemes delivered. Rather, they provided hospitals with a pool of nurses, guaranteed to be trained to the required standard, from which they could select the very best for the small number of staff vacancies. The situation in hospitals was quite different from that in offices, where managers expected all female workers to leave to be married, and could replace them with similarly skilled women instantly. In hospitals, the best nurses were the prized result of three years' nurturing. It seems unlikely that they would be happy to let nature (or fate) decide which nurses stayed and which left. At St George's, at least, the majority of nurses who failed to find a staff position at the end of training, moved to other nursing jobs – often in new sectors – indicating their desire to experience other forms of nursing, and to build up what would now be described as a portfolio of skills.

A final point is worth making on the 'inevitability' of marriage. While this was undoubtedly the case for many young women, the relatively low levels of marriage amongst its nurses, suggests that St George's (at least) attracted a very different group of women from those who rushed into offices. Vicinus and others have suggested that the desire for a husband among Victorian women was perhaps not as ubiquitous as has traditionally been believed (Vicinus 1985; A Vickery 1998). Far from finding themselves alone and discarded, some deliberately chose not to marry, preferring independence to a life confined by traditional Victorian family values. For such women, nursing could offer precisely the independence and self-determination they craved.

In examining the women who chose nursing as a career, as opposed to other options available to them at the time, it seems that it offered a very positive choice. That women were making this choice later in life than those who chose shop or office work, suggests that it was a more considered choice; and in light of the benefits nursing could offer (a reasonable wage, a set of skills highly valued by employers and society, promotion, and the chance for independence and travel) it does not seem the strange choice that Christopher Maggs struggled with (1980). The initial three years may have been far from pleasant, but they held out the opportunity for single women to be financially and personally independent, a very rare situation for Victorian women, even at the end of the century. The women who chose nursing – at St George's at least – exhibited such determination; and their decisions appear to have been driven as much by a need (or desire) to earn their own living, as through any other motivation.

The findings of this study are echoed in the challenges faced by nursing today. The relationship between medicine and nursing and the struggles over territory are as familiar now as they were in the nineteenth century. The deskilling of tasks (which began with the transfer of temperature-taking from doctors to nurses) continued into the twentieth century, ensuring that nursing as an occupation was kept subordinate to medicine. Nurses continue to take on tasks considered to be tedious or routine by their medical colleagues, and the fact that nurses provide a cheaper form of labour cannot be overlooked. Equally, they continue to fight for increased responsibility in the provision of healthcare, as demonstrated by their willingness to adopt 'nurse consultant' and 'nurse prescriber' roles. In such areas where nurses are perceived to have overstepped their natural boundaries, the medical profession is quick to mount an attack, branding them second-class practitioners and accusing them of endangering the care of patients.

This study has provided strong challenges to several assumptions concerning Victorian nurses. It has reaffirmed the conclusions of historians such as Maggs and Williams that the evidence left by nurse leaders cannot be assumed to represent the reality of being a nurse in the nineteenth century; but has gone further in postulating a much stronger character for many nurses. Women who entered nursing made a positive and informed decision to do so, and it is argued here, that they did so with the intention of making it a career, rather than as a stop-gap before marriage. The use of a novel methodology, which marries archival and census records in order to build biographical details of individual nurses, has revealed – for the first time – the detailed working of a nursing department in a large Victorian teaching hospital, and the lives of the women who worked in its wards.

Pen Portrait 6 Florence Smedley – innovative nurse educator

Florence Smedley revolutionized nurse training at two London hospitals. She epitomized the 'modern nurse' of late nineteenth-century England. Born to a wealthy family in 1856, she entered St Bartholomew's (Bart's) as a probationer in 1884 at the age of 28. This was an exciting time for nursing at Bart's. Ethel Manson (later Fenwick), newly appointed Matron, was overhauling nurse training. Florence thrived on nursing. In 1887, she passed her exams, finishing joint top of the list, and won a Gold Medal. Her stay at Bart's, as ward sister, lasted six years; and she developed the reputation for being a good organizer and 'excellent teacher' (*NR*, 21 April 1894: 264). In 1893, she moved to a convalescent home at Swanley to become Matron. Here she was able to develop her own ideas about nursing. Less than a year later, she was appointed Lady Superintendent at the Hospital for Sick Children at Great Ormond Street (HSC).

At the HSC Florence was able to put her ideas on nursing into practice. She found nurse training in a state of turmoil, after several failed attempts by previous matrons to introduce rigour and structure into a scheme which lacked both. Immediately, she launched a vigorous campaign for examinations and a timetable for lectures and practical instruction. She bombarded the board with letters, demands and instructions as to what should be done. By the time she left, the Nursing Department had been completely overhauled.

In 1897, St George's (looking to replace their long-serving Matron, Harriet Coster) chose Florence Smedley from a field of 37 candidates. *Nursing Record* applauded the decision, noting 'it is the more satisfactory because it is an open secret that ... strenuous efforts were made to [elect] a person whose professional record has been so questionable' (*NR*, 5 June 1897: 458). Florence found the situation to be even more dire than that at the HSC, and deluged the managers with reform after reform. They were overwhelmed by her energy, and most of her demands were met. The list of innovations she brought to St George's was legion: she took direct control of probationer training; introduced a timetable for lectures and practical instruction; limited entry to the scheme to set times during the year; introduced sisters from other hospitals, more rigorous rules for all nurses, a formal pension scheme and a four-year probationer contract. By the end of the nineteenth century the Nursing Department was unrecognizable from Mrs Coster's time, and bore close resemblance to that at the HSC and Bart's.

For all her vigour within the hospital, Florence Smedley did not participate in the public debate on nursing. But like the majority of her colleagues at London hospitals, it seems she opposed nurse registration: her name appearing in a list of signatures to the 1904 'antiregistrationist manifesto' published in *Nursing Record* (*NR*, 16 April 1904: 372).

Sadly, Florence was forced to retire from St George's in 1907, after a protracted and serious illness. She died in 1934.

Appendix 1
Methodology

A paucity of evidence from ordinary working women in the Victorian period makes it necessary to seek alternative sources to uncover their lives. This study has developed prosopographical techniques to build an understanding of a group of nurses who worked at St George's Hospital, London, in the period 1850–1900.

The technique of prosopography has been defined by Lawrence Stone as the 'investigation of the common background characteristics of a group of actors in history by means of a collective study of their lives' (1971: 46). At its root, prosopography provides a methodology for bringing together incomplete facts from diverse sources to create a whole. It has several applications in history, but the one most pertinent to this study relates to its use in studying social mobility and composition of a particular occupation, in this case, nursing.

The technique has its limitations: quality and quantity of data available, difficulties in linking disparate data fragments to a single individual, and potential errors in data interpretation are challenging. In this study, while the 1850–1900 dataset is large, individual datasets for the 1850s and 1860s are relatively small, making analysis in this period problematic. Presence of inherent biases in small datasets, which can produce unrepresentative results, must be identified: in this study, for example, matrons appeared easier to track in the various sources than ordinary nurses. Their presence may have skewed class composition of the Nursing Department in favour of the higher classes in earlier decades. Despite these drawbacks, if used with caution, the technique can uncover information previously thought impossible to retrieve.

Sources used in this study have been described in the Introduction. The Nurse Registers formed the major source. They were kept in bound books, with pre-printed column headings: Table A1.1 describes their content and the frequency with which information was recorded.

Information for years prior to 1869 was extracted from the Weekly Board and Committee of Nursing minutes, and a set of Wage Books from 1849 to 1860. All data were entered into a Microsoft Access database (the St George's Hospital Nurses' Database) in a series of tables relating to the

Table A1.1 Content of St George's Hospital Nurse Registers (1870–1900)

920 individual nurses	%
Name	100
Age at start	98
Previous occupation	96
Date of start	100
Date left	88
Reasons for leaving	89
Promotions and exams passed	45
Father's occupation	24
Subsequent employment	11
Contact address	12

Source: Hawkins 2010.

original source. Record linkage techniques were used to link multiple entries for the same individual based on common name, dates, roles and wards worked on. The process of record linkage in historical research is well documented (see for instance French and Tilley 1997).

While the hospital archive contained plentiful information on nurses at the hospital, their lives before and after were not well documented. The census returns for 1841–1901 were used to fill in these gaps.

Of 431 individual nurses identified in the hospital census returns (1841 to 1901), 52 per cent were traced in other censuses, providing information on family life before entering the hospital and their fate after leaving. (A commercial online census service – Ancestry.com – was used for this study.). To identify records between censuses, matches on three main characteristics were required: name, place of birth and age. The pitfalls of using censuses to identify individuals are well known: errors in collection, inconsistent ages and place of birth between censuses, and misspelling of unusual names can be added to errors in transcription both at the time, and in the modern day (Higgs 2005). In this study a match required an exact match, or understandable mutation, of the name, a place of birth within close proximity to the original entry, and a date of birth within five years of expected date.

The occupation information from the censuses enabled analysis of the class structure of St George's Nursing Department. The use of census data to study the social structure of Victorian society has a long history. Walter Armstrong has discussed the challenges in using it in this way, and has developed a system for the assignment of class based on census occupation data (1972). He has adapted the 1950 Registrar General's classification of occupations to reflect Victorian occupations, and their implied social status for this purpose. His scheme has been adopted by many social historians. Mills and Schurer have discussed the merits of various schemes for classifying Victorian occupations and claim Armstrong's method has 'won

Table A1.2 Occupations and class

Class	Typical occupations
Class I (upper and middle class)	Military officers; doctors; clergymen; accountants; museum curators; surveyors; architects; business owners
Class II (intermediate class)	Teachers; Inland Revenue collectors; veterinary surgeons; land agents; railway inspectors; stationmasters; farmers; manufacturers; larger shop-owners and lodging-house proprietors
Class III (skilled working class)	Artisans (e.g. lace-makers; carpenters; builders; etc.); tradesmen (e.g. grocers; stationers; dressmakers; etc.); smaller shop owners and lodging house proprietors
Class IV (semi-skilled working class)	Domestic servants; brickmakers; gardeners
Class V (unskilled working class)	Labourers; porters

Source: Armstrong 1972.

substantial support from students of the census' (1996: 152). For the purposes of comparison, if no other, they recommend that any, 'serious study of social stratification should make use of it' (1996: 152). Armstrong's scheme was therefore selected for use in this study. His class structure and sample occupations are listed in Table A1.2.

Several occupations are problematic. Social class of farmers, manufacturers and lodging-house keepers depends on the size of their enterprise. Armstrong places all farmers in Class II, but this may be inappropriate. In the St George's dataset, farmers' daughters came from enterprises ranging from 11 acres to over 500 acres. In this study, size of farm has dictated class, to a limited extent, with the smallest taken as belonging to Class III (Mills 1999). With manufacturers and lodging-house keepers, the size of the workforce is critical. Armstrong suggests that shop-owners, lodging-house keepers, merchants and dealers employing one or more people (excluding family members and domestic servants) should be placed in Class II. This advice was followed. If no information was available on number of employees, the individuals were placed in Class III.

In the majority of cases, the women were initially found as children in the family home, and class was assigned based on the father's occupation. If the father was absent or dead, the mother's occupation (if she had one) was used. Where the first trace of a woman occurred after she had left home, her own occupation was taken as an indicator of her social class. Widows were assigned a class based on their husband's occupation.

Table A1.3 Database statistics

Named nurses in database	1,473
Nurses with length of service detail	1,062
Nurses where place and date of birth is known	453
Nurses with class assigned	350
Nurses whose occupation before St George's is known	991
Nurses with full or part careers documented	120

The resulting combination of data from the censuses and various archival records has enabled a detailed and unique database of nurses' lives to be constructed (see Table A1.3). The numbers of women thus traced have enabled this unique study of a nursing department, during a period of significant development for the profession as a whole.

Appendix 2

Comparison of nursing departments at 12 London hospitals, 1890s

Table A2.1

Hospital	Type/year founded*	Number of beds	Size of Nursing Dept.	Paying probationers	Private nursing institution	Beds : nurses ratio**	Length of probation***	Accommodation#	Matron
St Bartholomew's	Endowed, 1123	674	238	Yes	Yes	2.2	4 years (ordinary) 3 months (paying)	Bedrooms	Isla Stewart
St Thomas'	Endowed, 1228	569*	142	Yes*	No	2.5	4 years	Separate bedrooms (paying pros)	Miss Gordon
Guy's	Endowed, 1721	690*	119	Yes*	Yes	2.3	3 years (ordinary) 1 year (paying)	Cubicles	Miss Nott Bower*
The London	Voluntary, 1740	770*	245*	Yes*	Yes	2.3	3 years (ordinary) 3 months (paying)	Separate bedrooms	Miss Luckes

Hospital	Foundation						Training		Matron
The Middlesex	Voluntary, 1745	321	102	Yes	Yes	3	1 year (ordinary) 6–12 months (paying)	Cubicles	Miss Thorold
Charing Cross	Voluntary, 1834	175	82	Yes		2.6	3 years (ordinary) 1 year (paying)		Miss H Gordon*
The Westminster	Voluntary, 1719	205*	57*	No*	Yes	4.6			Miss Pyne*
St George's	Voluntary, 1733	351	118	No	No	2.5	3 years	Cubicles	Mrs Coster
University College Hospital	Voluntary, 1833	207*	90*			2.1	3 years		Sister Cecilia*
King's College Hospital	Voluntary, 1839	220	73	Yes	Yes	2.3	3 years		Miss Monk*
St Mary's	Voluntary, 1851	281	65	Yes	No	3.7	3 years (ordinary) 1 year (paying)		Miss Medill*
The Royal Free	Voluntary, 1828	166	39	Yes	No	2.6	4 years (ordinary) 6 months (paying)		Miss Wedgewood

Sources: Charles Booth Archive (1896) except where indicated otherwise; * The Nursing Record 6 October 1894, pp. 217–28; ** The Hospital (Nursing Mirror Supplement) 2 November 1895, p. 85; *** The Hospital (Nursing Mirror Supplement) commencing 1 August 1896; # Morten 1892

Appendix 3

Sample occupations of fathers (or mothers) of St George's nurses

Class I

Accountant
Army officer
Bank manager
Business owner
Churchman
Commissioner, Indian Civil Service
Company director
Doctor
Gentleman farmer
Independent
Inland Revenue officer
Land-owner
Lawyer
Surveyor

Class II

Book-keeper
Corn-merchant
Farmer
Manager of factory/mill
Merchant
Small business owner
Stationmaster
Ship's captain
Teacher
Veterinary surgeon

Class III

Baker
Bootmaker

Bricklayer
Butcher
Carpenter
Clerk
Cooper
Decorator
Engine driver
Factory foreman
Gamekeeper
Greengrocer
Mechanic
Musician
Needlewoman
Plumber
Policeman
Saddler
Shipsmith
Stonemason
Tailor
Traveller
Watchmaker
Weaver

Class IV

Agricultural labourer
Brickburner
Cow-keeper
Gardener
Horse-keeper
Railway worker
Servant

Class V

Labourer
Railway porter

Notes

Introduction: constructing new nursing and a new history of nursing

1 Ethel Fenwick is usually referred to by historians as Mrs Bedford Fenwick, but she only used her husband's full name, in an official capacity, when she was working for the *Nursing Record*. On all other official occasions (particularly those connected to the Royal British Nursing Association) she referred to herself as Ethel Gordon Fenwick (Brooks and Rafferty 2007). In this book, she will be referred to as Ethel Fenwick throughout.

2 Student nurses continued to be exhorted to derive inspiration from an heroic past, as the following passage from nursing textbook illustrates: 'An understanding of the historical traditions, ideals of service, and Christian principles of those who have gone before them is the rightful inheritance of all nurses and will add dignity and meaning to their work' (Jamieson *et al.* 1966).

3 'History from below' focuses on the perspective of ordinary individuals within society or the section of society under study (Evans 2000). It is often used to study groups previously ignored by historians, such as women and the working classes, and as such, is an extremely useful tool for the study of nurses.

4 In this period UCH was nursed by the All Saints Sisterhood, one of several organizations of Anglican women which emerged in the mid-nineteenth century to provide nursing care to the poor. Anne Summers has written extensively on the subject (Summers 1991).

5 *An Introduction to the Social History of Nursing* (1988) remains a landmark in nursing history, and the authors' consideration of external influences on nursing set a standard by which other nurse historians can be measured.

6 Thetis Group and Joan Roberts have suggested that feminists should reappraise Nightingale, by shifting the focus away from her nursing reforms (which fit neatly into the feminine 'Victorian Lady' stereotype) to her achievements in the 'male' sphere, as a medical statistician, reformer of the British Army Medical Corps, political expert on India and creator of the Indian Sanitary Commission (Group and Roberts 2001).

7 The Sairey Gamp character, in Charles Dickens' novel *Martin Chuzzlewit*, was depicted as 'slovenly, dirty and boozy' monthly nurse.

8 According to the British Library catalogue, 40 books on Nightingale have been published since 1990, five in 2009; and with the centenary of her death in 2010, a slew of new works on this venerable lady can be expected.

9 Such nurse historians include, among others, Christine Hallett, Stephanie Kirby, Helen Sweet, Barbara Mortimer, Stuart Wildman and Susan McGann, who have addressed a wide range of topics and raised the importance of rigorous methodology in nursing history.

10 The *International History of Nursing Journal* ceased publication in 2003 when *Nursing Standard* withdrew its support.

11 Prosopography is a methodology which enables 'the investigation of the common background characteristics of a group of actors in history by means of a collective study of their lives' (Stone 1971: 46). The database is referred to throughout as the 'St George's Hospital Nurses Database' (SGHNDB). The methodology used in this study is described in detail in Appendix 1.

12 Ann Digby and John Stewart have described the technique of prosopography as a, 'useful approach in analysing the dynamics of group agency', through which 'family background, education, social or political philosophy, career aspiration … [become] highly visible' (Digby and Stewart 1996: 14). Julia Parker and Jane Lewis have used the technique to study groups of female reformers. (Parker 1988; Lewis 1991).

13 The 1861 census for St George Hanover Square, in which the hospital was located, was destroyed by fire in the mid-twentieth century and was therefore not available for this study.

14 These interviews are discussed in Chapter 2. The Booth Collection is housed at The British Library of Political and Economic Science (the Library of the London School of Economics and Political Science). The catalogue is available online at http://booth.lse.ac.uk/ (accessed on 28 July 2009).

1 The search for self-esteem

1 Three notable exceptions to this are St Thomas', St Bartholomew's and Guy's, which were financed by large endowments.

2 Trudgill acknowledges that by the nineteenth century such sentiments were less likely to be spoken directly, but were still commonly held, among nineteenth-century men.

3 This element of respectability also spread among the working classes, putting pressure on the wives of members of the 'labour aristocracy' (at least) to refrain from paid work on pain of loss of respectability (Rose 1992).

4 Kamchatka is a peninsula in the far east of Russia.

5 By 1885 there were still only 50 female guardians in the whole system. Numbers began to rise in the mid-1890s, after the abolition of the property qualification for candidates, and by 1910 there were over 1,600 female Poor Law guardians (King 2006).

6 The Alexandra Hip Hospital was such an exception, founded by Catherine Wood and Miss Spencer Percival, nurses from nearby Great Ormond Street Hospital (HSC). The HSC itself maintained an all-male board of management throughout the nineteenth century. (Alexandra Hospital for Children with Hip Disease 2007).

7 The Women's Hospital in Nottingham is another exception. It was managed on a day-to-day basis by a committee of ladies for 20 years. The weekly committee was overseen by a quarterly committee which included '12 gentlemen' in addition to the ladies (Taylor 1997).

8 This analogy was also used to reduce the inherent dangers of intimacy between the male patient and female nurse. By rendering the male patient as a child, the sexual nature of the contact between the two was alleviated, to a certain extent.

9 Catherine Judd has highlighted how this strategy rebounded on nurse reformers; the very image which they created of saintly nurses was heavily steeped in sexual fantasy, and a symbol of yet another Victorian dichotomy, this time, nurse as saintly Madonna and seductive Magdalen (1998).

10 St John's House Sisterhood was one of the first Protestant nursing sisterhoods, along with Elizabeth Fry's Institute of Nursing Sisters (founded in 1840), to be

founded in England. Unlike Fry's organization, which focused on home
nursing, one its first objectives was to form connections with hospitals (Moore
1988).

11 An upsurge in the formation of English Catholic female congregations, in the
early part of the nineteenth century, enabled Catholic women to combine deep
religiosity with work amongst the sick poor (Mangion 2008). This movement
may have offered a model for their Protestant sisters, also searching for an
outlet for religiously motivated philanthropy.

12 Although their presence in the large hospitals dwindled, the nursing sisterhoods continued to work among the poor in their homes (Sweet and Dougal
2008).

13 Simonton and Verslusyen have both proposed that Nightingale's conflation of
a good woman with a good nurse has been at the root of difficulties in gaining
respect for nursing as a profession. It left many aspects of nursing too closely
associated with the natural domestic role of women, deskilling it, and ensuring
a nurse's authority derived only from her relationship with male authority
(Simonton 2001; Versluysen 1980).

14 In the Victorian psyche, poverty, disease and sin were all inextricably inter-
twined, and a hospital, which brought all three together in a single location,
was a very dangerous place (Bashford 1998; Judd 1998).

15 The reaction of doctors to the introduction of middle-class nurses is discussed
in detail in Chapter 3.

16 A profession must have four basic attributes: a body of knowledge which it lays
exclusive claim to, formalized training and tests of proficiency, regulation of its
practices by a professional association, and restricted entry (Abbott 1988; Corfield 1995). Nurses, in demanding access to the medical curriculum, were
threatening the first of these.

17 The anomaly was pointed out by one of Fenwick's most ardent critics, Henry
Burdett, who expressed surprise that a 'nurse-led' movement had 100 medical
men on its general council and 14 doctors on the executive committee (*H/NM*,
17 March 1888).

18 For a detailed discussion of the battle for registration see, for example, Dingwall *et al.* 1988.

19 In a recent example, the chairman of the BMA Consultants' Committee
described the introduction of nurse prescribers as 'an irresponsible and dangerous move. ... Patients will suffer. I would not have me or my family subject
to anything other than highest level of care ... which is provided by a fully
trained doctor' (Miller 2005).

20 On the general problem of 'surplus women' see Holcombe 1973 or Poovey
1989. On the link between the 'surplus women' problem and the development
of the new nurse, see Simonton 2001; Dingwall *et al.* 1988; Vicinus 1985.

21 The number of unmarried women continued to grow throughout the rest of
the century, such that by the time of the 1911 census, there were over 1.4
million more women than men in England (Holcombe 1973).

22 Founded in 1859, the Society for Promoting the Employment of Women
(SPEW) aimed to reform women's social position through improved education
and employment opportunities (Tusan 2000).

23 A good example of the pressure to postpone marriage can be found in a collection of letters, between Adrian Hope and Laura Troubridge, charting the
course of their long engagement in the 1880s. Hope (secretary to the Hospital
for Sick Children) and his fiancée were obliged, through lack of money, to
prolong their engagement for four years. In December 1887, Laura wrote, 'I
cannot marry you dearest until you are free from debts. ... Is there no chance
of your salary at Great O. St being raised?' (Lancaster 2002: 399).

24 Florence Nightingale is a good example of a woman desperate to escape the tedium of home life and the threat of its perpetuation in marriage. Other women who chose spinsterhood include feminists Frances Power Cobbe, Emily Davies (founder of Girton College, Cambridge), and Emily Rayner Parkes and Jessie Boucherett, members of the Langham Place group (Deane 1996).

25 Nightingale, Twining and the feminists of Langham Place all fit into this category. Notable exceptions include Harriet Martineau, obliged to support herself through her writing, and Octavia Hill who worked as a secretary for at least part of her life (Webb 2006; Darley 2006).

2 'The majority are ladies, a great many domestics'

1 Booth B153 (Carwen), p. 60, 8 April 1896.

2 Parents of patients at the Hospital for Sick Children (HSC) greeted the introduction of lady nurses enthusiastically: 'it is different now that there is a lady out there … no favours … it's quite the talk among us poor folk in London, if we were ladies we cd [*sic*] not be better treated' (GOS5/2/30, 13 May 1875).

3 Maggs coined the term from evidence given to the 1904 House of Commons Select Committee on the Registration of Nurses.

4 Most of Maggs' evidence on class in Victorian nursing was drawn from two sources: Mary H. Annesley Voysey, *Nursing: hints to probationers on practical work*, London: Scientific Press, 1905; and *Report from the Select Committee on the Registration of Nurses*, London: HMSO, 1904.

5 Figure 2.1 was created using the data in Simnet's paper and the methodology described in Appendix 1 of this study, enabling direct comparisons between the nursing departments of Bart's and St George's (Simnet 1986).

6 The system at St Thomas' combined ordinary probationers (paid a small wage during training) with special probationers who paid for the privilege. The special probationer scheme was enormously successful, and large numbers of 'ladies' clamoured to be admitted, drawn by the aura surrounding Nightingale and her exploits in the Crimea (Parry and Parry 1976; Granshaw 1981; Baly 1987).

7 Rosalind Paget (1855–1948) was a trained midwife and campaigner for state control of midwifery. She came from a long line of social reformers, which included her uncle, William Rathbone (1819–1902), MP for Liverpool, who introduced a training school for district nurses in that city. Paget trained as a nurse at the Westminster Hospital and gained her diploma in midwifery from the London Obstetrical Society. The 1902 Midwives Act, which she was instrumental in pushing through, provided for registration and a central monitoring board, and outlawed the practice of midwifery without a certificate. Paget was also a strong supporter of women's suffrage (Hannam 2004a; Sweet and Dougal 2008).

8 Paget had a poor opinion of general nurses, regarding them as 'a discontented race'. She considered nursing to be 'exceedingly easy' compared with domestic service or shop work.

9 The editor of *The Hospital* was inundated with letters on this subject for a whole month and finally drew a line under any further discussion, stating he would not print any more on the subject (Editorial *H/NM*, 24 September 1898).

10 Isla Stewart (1856–1910) came from a solid middle-class background. Her father was a farmer and journalist, and she was educated by governesses at home. She trained at the Nightingale School, and after working at various hospitals was appointed Matron at Bart's in 1887. Stewart was a close ally of Ethel Fenwick in the registration debates; improving nurse education was her main priority (McGann 1992).

11 The growth in popularity of nurse training is discussed in more detail in Chapter 3.
12 The Nurses' Cooperation was a London-based private nursing institution. It is discussed in more detail in Chapter 4.
13 The QNI arose out of Lees' original London-based association in the 1880s.
14 For a discussion of the use of micro-history in a wider context see Hudson 1999.
15 In Simnet's study, for instance, the upper and middle classes already represented over 60 per cent of the annual intake of probationers by 1883 (1986).
16 Any subscriber of £5 annually or donor of £50 was eligible to take a seat on the Board and participate in the hospital's management.
17 The only resident officers were the Apothecary and the surgeon's apprentice. These rules indicate that the Matron's authority was subordinate to that of the Apothecary, who stood in lieu of the medical men (Blomfield 1933).
18 Blomfield claims the new hospital opened with 350 beds.
19 That recruits were expected to possess 'medical knowledge' is surprising, and contradicts the view of 'old style' nurses as being ignorant, although the nature of this knowledge was never discussed.
20 Fry's nurses had previously been trained at Guy's and the London, but the Society was looking to extend its hospital contacts.
21 This subject is discussed in Chapter 3.
22 The hospital continued to employ night nurses for several years after this (SGHWB/55, 19 April 1893).
23 According to Dent, the changes at St George's resulted from Nightingale's advice on hospital design (Dent 1894c). But not all commentators agreed with Nightingale. In 1863, Timothy Holmes and Dr J.S. Bristowe produced a report on the state of England's hospitals, which contradicted her ideas, both on the siting of hospitals and their construction (Woodward 1974).
24 'Hospital diseases', such as erysipelas, pyaemia and phagadaena, were the scourge of hospitalized patients, especially surgical cases (Woodward 1974).
25 For a discussion of the impact of germ theory on hospital design see Hayward 1998. For a modern discussion on hospitalism see Bynum 2001: 1372.
26 'Specials' were nurses working either independently or for private nursing institutions, and hired by the hospital on a temporary basis.
27 Male nurses (or attendants) were used where patients were violent, or posed a physical threat to female nurses, such as in cases of delirium tremens. At St George's, they were supplied by the Hamilton Nursing Association, one of the few male nursing agencies. There have been some studies on male asylum nurses, but little has been written about their counterparts in the voluntary sector. Arlene Young has discussed the subject briefly (2008), but it warrants further research.
28 Other imperatives behind the drive to increase probationer numbers (such as the demand for improved education) are discussed in Chapter 3, but clearly the financial benefits cannot be ignored.
29 Honnor Morten's *How to Become a Nurse and How to Succeed* was first printed in 1893, and by 1895 was on its third edition. Henry Burdett's *The Nursing Profession: how and where to train, being a guide to training for the profession of a nurse,* London: Scientific Press, was first published in 1899, and was republished in various forms up to 1933.
30 Such manuals were not exclusive to nursing. As occupations opened up to women in the late nineteenth century, so too did a new opportunity for publishers. Manuals offering advice for entry into a wide range of occupations began to appear: see for instance, James Graham's *The Beginners Guide to Office Work* published in 1898, Frances Low's *Press Work for Women: a textbook for the*

young women journalists, published in 1904, or John Newton's *How to Become a Pupil Teacher* from 1885.

31 The high turnover in nursing staff and the strategies adopted by the hospital for its management are discussed in detail in Chapter 4.

32 A detailed discussion of the methodology used in this study can be found in Appendix 1. Six of these profiles are distributed throughout this book.

33 Extracts from this discussion on the influence of social class on nurses' careers will appear in Hawkins 2010.

34 The data for 1842–51 were collected in a fortuitous way. In the 1851 census, the column headed 'Rank, Profession or Occupation' was completed incorrectly. The instructions for the column read 'State here the profession, or what is believed to have been the ordinary occupation of the Inmate before admission into the Institution' (Decennial Census 1851). While this was obviously intended to refer to the occupation of the patients only, the instruction was applied to all individuals in the return. Consequently, the previous profession of all the hospital's employees was recorded. This information would otherwise have been very difficult to trace, as the 1841 census (which would have been the primary source) provides only very limited information on place of birth and no information on family relationships.

35 This disadvantage of prosopography is discussed in detail in Appendix 1.

36 Where the first trace of a woman in the census occurred after she had already left home, her own occupation was taken as an indicator of her social class.

37 Women in these social classes needed to earn a living from a young age (either to support themselves or to contribute to the family finances). With several years elapsing before they could contemplate nursing (as a result of minimum age barriers), many were found in census returns living away from home, and were classified according to their own occupation, rather than that of their fathers.

38 The shared history of these two hospitals has already been discussed, and it is interesting to reflect on the impact of that shared history on the origins of this common, and unusual, characteristic.

39 The term 'lady nurses' is used throughout this book to refer to women who entered hospitals for a short period of time, to acquire rudimentary nursing skills, or who volunteered to work as nurses in hospitals. Paying probationers refers to women who paid to be included in a specific training scheme.

40 No note remains as to the identity of this woman. The 'lady nurses' in question at King's would have been members of the St John's House Sisterhood, which had recently taken over the nursing of the hospital (Moore 1988).

41 The expectation that middle-class nurses would provide moral leadership within hospitals is discussed in Chapter 1.

42 Advertisements were placed in *The Times* soliciting donations from the general public, and a collector was appointed to visit the 'gentry and nobility' in the hospital's immediate vicinity to gain subscriptions.

43 The monthly wage bill for the Nursing Department was in the region of £350, or £4,260 a year, making it a very vulnerable target for cost-cutting exercises (SGHWB/31, 26 September 1860).

44 According to Helmstadter, it was the open nature of St George's Weekly Board which concerned the St John's Sisters (C. Helmstadter, personal communication, 2007).

45 This ad hoc committee became the Committee for Nursing, in April 1868. It comprised representatives of the institution's officers (the treasurer, physicians, surgeons and the visiting apothecaries) and ten governors. The Matron was not included, but was invited to attend as an ex officio member (SGHWB/33, 24 January 1866 and 21 February 1866).

46 St Peter's House (or St Peter's Home, as it was also called) was an Anglican sisterhood, established by Benjamin Lancaster – a governor of St George's – and his wife Rosamira and supported by the Bishop of London. Opened in 1861, in Brompton Square, the home was to provide convalescent care for patients discharged from the hospital. It later moved to Kilburn, north London ('Community of St Peter, Kilburn, Woking and elsewhere', n.d.).

47 The debate within the committee of St George's presaged similar, but more public, disputes which erupted at King's in the early 1870s, when doctors accused the nurses (members of the St John's Sisterhood) of being 'more loyal to the Order than to the hospital or its staff' (Waddington 1995: 219).

48 Dr Charles West, founder of the Hospital for Sick Children at Great Ormond Street, used the same argument against a similar experiment at his own hospital: 'Sooner or later religious difficulty will occur ... Some of the supporters of the Hospital will take exception to this or that practice either of so-called High or Low Church; for on both sides the danger is equal' (GOS/11/1/10, 20 January 1876).

49 Lady visitors to the hospital are discussed in more detail in Chapter 1.

50 Initial use of the term 'lady' conveyed a set of attributes which the governors expected their new matron to possess, and which would distinguish her from matrons of the past. The decision to abandon its use found echoes in the hospital's long avoidance of the title 'sister' for the heads of wards. If the aversion to 'sister' can be explained by a desire to appear to be secular, perhaps the avoidance of 'lady' indicates a similar desire not to be seen as elitist?

51 At St Thomas' lady pupils attended special lectures (Granshaw 1981). Bart's had a special home for lady probationers (Morten 1892); the Middlesex excused them 'menial tasks', while the London excused them night duty (*NR*, 6 October 1894: 213–18).

52 Charles Hawkins was a 'pre-eminent figure on the Board of Governors' of St George's Hospital, being Treasurer from 1865 to 1870. Although he had failed to be elected to the medical staff during the 1840s, he continued to dedicate his life to the hospital as a governor. He was a member of the Council of the Royal College of Surgeons (Gould and Uttley 1997).

53 According to the Matron, Emily Jones 'was suffering from some dreadful delusion, rendering her residence in the Hospital impossible' (SGHCON/1, 18 November 1868).

54 Zepharina Veitch (1836–94) was the elder daughter of William Douglas Veitch, vicar of St Saviour's Paddington, from whom she inherited a passion for social welfare reform. After leaving St George's she rejoined the All Saints Sisters to travel to Sedan during the Franco-Prussian war and on her return, she trained as a midwife and campaigned for the improvement of midwives' training. She married surgeon Henry Smith in 1876 and although she stopped practising, she continued to fight for reform. Veitch was one of the founder members, and later President, of the Midwives Institute. Her colleague Rosalind Paget described her book, *A Handbook for Nursing the Sick*, as the best book on nursing ever written (Hannam 2004b).

55 Veitch was anxious to protest her innocence of the charge of ritualism, a term used to describe members of the Church of England who followed doctrines more closely allied to the Catholic church, such as transubstantiation and the sacrament of the confession (Ryle *c.*1870).

56 This period of the hospital's history is discussed in more depth in Chapter 4.

57 See Pen Portrait 1 (p. 34), for a brief biography of Harriet Coster.

58 See Pen Portrait 6 (p. 183) for a brief biography of Florence Smedley.

59 Four of the sisters appointed by Miss Smedley had trained either at the HSC or

at Bart's, demonstrating the importance of networks in building careers, and also in consolidating authority.

60 According to F.M.L. Thompson, by the mid-nineteenth century the mean age for marriage for women was 25, and remained at this level for the rest of the century (1988: 52). Joan Perkin assigned an average age of marriage between 23 and 26 for all classes of women (1993: 2).

61 One of Harriet Coster's children was allowed to live in her mother's rooms on several occasions when she was seriously ill (SGHCON/2, 11 January 1892; SGHWB/55, 23 November 1892).

62 See Pen Portrait 3 (p. 108) for an example for a nurse who probably concealed her status as a mother from the authorities.

63 The 1841 census did not record place of birth, but merely indicated if the person was born in the same county as the place of the census. In this census, 30 per cent of nurses at St George's were born in Middlesex.

3 Probationer schemes: education or cheap labour?

1 Baly has suggested that Nightingale considered theoretical knowledge of secondary importance compared to moral and character training. Her continued rejection of the germ theory, and antagonism toward the examination of nurses, are cited in support of this argument (Baly 1987). Bradshaw, who regards such historians as 'revisionist', counters that this is to misunderstand Nightingale, who, she claims, supported both elements of nurse training, in equal balance (2000).

2 The growth in interest in further education among young middle-class women has been discussed in Chapter 1, and it was this trend which nurse leaders were hoping to bend to their advantage when planning more formal training schemes.

3 While some women did take up apprenticeships in the tailoring trade, their numbers were insignificant in comparison to those who worked in unskilled, piecework.

4 Wood wrote extensively about teaching nurses to make best use of their inherent skills, for example in a series of articles in *Nursing Record* in 1888 on the training of nurses for sick children.

5 The Female Medical Society was founded, in 1862, along with its sister organization, the Ladies' Medical College, whose objective was to train female midwives and doctors. The college had some limited success before its activities were eclipsed by the opening of the London School of Medicine for Women, by Sophia Jex-Blake, in 1874 (Parry and Parry 1976; Blake 1990).

6 See Edward Domville's *Manual for Hospital Nurses and Others Engaged in Caring for the Sick*, published in 1888, or C.S. Weekshaw and William Radford's, *A Text-Book of Nursing* published in 1897. A review of a wide range of nineteenth-century nursing textbooks reveals that messages concerning the moral character and ethos of nursing were repeated over and over again (Bradshaw 2000).

7 Anne Marie Rafferty has argued that nurse leaders, such as Ethel Fenwick, deliberately adopted elements of the medical curriculum as part of a wider strategy to emulate the doctors' own bid for registration, based on the assumption that a strategy that had been proved to work for one group would be likely to succeed for another (Rafferty 1996).

8 Miasmatic theory of infection connected disease with dirt and ultimately with sin. In Nightingale's eyes it was the role of the nurse to place a patient in 'the best condition for nature to act upon him', and this included care of the spiritual as well as the physical environment (Nightingale 1861).

9 Catherine Wood encouraged nurses to ask questions and learn from experience, 'to build [their] own knowledge, not get it ready made' (Bradshaw 2000: 8).

10 The hospital's role as medical laboratory was widely acknowledged. The Hospital for Sick Children at Great Ormond Street (HSC) included 'the attainment and diffusion of knowledge regarding the diseases of children' among its key objectives (GOS/1/1 1852–3).

11 According to sociologists, one of the key characteristics which distinguishes a profession from an occupation is tight control over membership, and nineteenth-century doctors jealously guarded entry to their profession (Abbott 1988).

12 Two influential medical members of the Royal British Nurses' Association (Dyce Duckworth, physician to St Bartholomew's, and Sir James Crichton-Browne, a Fellow of the Royal Society) both spoke out against the over-education of women from social Darwinist principles (Rafferty 1996; Allen 2001).

13 The Medical Registration Act of 1858 had unified the three branches of medicine (surgeons, physicians and apothecaries) and marked a legal closure of the profession, under the watchful eye of the newly formed General Medical Council (Parry and Parry 1976).

14 This female trait of patience and attention to detail was made much of in other areas of women's work. Female telegraphers 'bore long confinement with more patience' than their male counterparts (Davin 2005: 211), while women were 'temperamentally better suited to routine clerical work' (Holcombe 1973: 146). They were urged to stand as parish councillors, because they were 'so much more earnest about small things … and parish council work deals with matters of seemingly small import'; while Octavia Hill (social reformer), speaking on women's involvement in housing projects, declared 'ladies must do it for it is detailed work' (Digby 1992: 202–3).

15 Dr Steele (Medical Superintendent at Guy's in the late 1880s) reported that much of the increased workload of nurses (the subject of public debate at the time) resulted from the transfer of such cases to them from medical students (quoted in Anon. 1887).

16 The nurses' school at Bart's did not open until 1877 (Yeo 1995), classes for nurses first appeared at the London in 1881 (Clark-Kennedy 1962–3); and modernization of the Guy's nursing department began in 1879, with the appointment of Margaret Burt, a St John's House nurse, as Matron (Moore 1988). In the provinces, hospitals were more progressive. While not necessarily establishing training schools for some time, they were keen to employ women who had trained at St Thomas' or with one of the sisterhoods. Manchester Royal Infirmary sent an official to London in the early 1860s to investigate nurse training at St Thomas', King's and the Nursing Sisterhood Institute. He was to report on the feasibility of introducing a similar scheme in Manchester, and to find a suitably qualified lady to run it (MRIWB, October 1864). Institutions in the Midlands sent similar delegations, with the same purpose (Wildman 2007).

17 The Nightingale Fund (created from public donations during the Crimean War) was to be used to set up a school for nursing, and St Thomas' was selected to host the school. The fund covered each probationer's board and lodging and £10 salary. According to Monica Baly, St Thomas' only agreed to the experiment as a result of these financial incentives. This motive was further revealed when the hospital pressed for the number of probationers to be increased (Baly 1997).

18 A matron at one Birmingham hospital claimed (in 1887) that she could save £90 a year by hiring six probationers in place of five nurses (Wildman 2003).

19 The fees at St Thomas' were considerably lower, at £30 a year (Morten 1892).

20 This event has already been discussed in detail in Chapter 2.

21 Nine probationers were recruited during the first year of the scheme. Three had previous nursing experience, two had worked as laundresses and two as ladies' companions. The majority, therefore, appear to be of a similar background to the existing staff (SGHNDB).

22 Dr James Phillips Kay was a mid-nineteenth-century educational reformer. The quote comes from his influential book, *The Moral and Physical Condition of Working Classes Employed in the Cotton Manufacture in Manchester*, London, 1832.

23 The hospital's interest in its patients' spiritual well-being is displayed in the 1856 Annual Report: 'The patients are all supplied with Bibles ... during their residence. ... It is hoped ... [the hospital] may be made instrumental in imparting to them the knowledge of the Gospel.' The proximity of nurses to the patients lent them a special opportunity to support these objectives (*SGHAR* 1856: 22).

24 Examination of the hospital's accounts has revealed no income streams associated with nurse training.

25 This is the same Mrs Lancaster, whose husband petitioned the hospital some years later to take over the Nursing Department, using nurses from their own institution, St Peter's House.

26 The hospital had an ambivalent attitude to nursing sisterhoods, as has already been observed in their negotiations with St Peter's House. It had previously accepted several nursing sisters from East Grinstead to train, but this time the refusal was outright.

27 She may have been a daughter of Willem Frederick, Baron d'Ablaing van Giessenburg, a member of the Dutch aristocracy (World Roots Website, online).

28 It is possible that the record of lady nurses was kept in a separate series of registers which have not survived, but the extent of the surviving nursing records at St George's tends argue against this.

29 The phenomenon of sulky and surly special probationers lends support to arguments, frequently made in the nursing press, that some women were signing up with motives other than becoming a trained nurse, as discussed in Chapter 5.

30 Tensions between lady pupils and regular probationers at St Thomas' were well known. According to Lindsay Granshaw, by the end of the nineteenth century, they had reached such a pitch that the two-tier system had almost disappeared (Granshaw 1981).

31 This was an incredibly large amount of money for a woman to find, equivalent to nearly two years' wages for a probationer.

32 Other elements of the same plan (such as increased numbers of established staff and a reduction in probationers) never materialized. By the end of the year, the number of probationers had actually risen. The Weekly Board regularly returned to the question of organization of its Nursing Department and the minutes are full of plans which never left the drawing board. This may have been one of them.

33 The hospital made Nightingale an honorary governor in July 1856, and, according to Clinton Dent, she became the first Lady Governor of any hospital (Dent 1894c).

34 Carol Helmstadter has claimed that it was the doctors who 'led the push' for nurse education at St George's. This study has not uncovered unequivocal proof for this statement, but some evidence does support that interpretation (2002).

35 Edward Domville was surgeon to the Devon and Exeter Hospital and lecturer and examiner to the St John's Ambulance Association.

36 *Domville's* was one of the manuals Bradshaw consulted, but in her analysis she overlooked how different it was from the others in her collection. Of the 17 she reviewed, six were written by nurse leaders, three at least (Luckes, Wood and Nightingale) well known for their dedication to a Christian ethos. Two were written by doctors (Domville's *Manual for Hospital Nurses* and L. Humphry's *A Manual of Nursing*). Neither of these contained the sentiments expressed in the nurse-written manuals.

37 St Mary's, the Middlesex, and Charing Cross were the others mentioned in the article.

38 This is discussed in more detail in Chapter 4.

39 The strong influence of medical men on the general management of St George's was quite unusual. But given that it was founded by the breakaway medical faculty of the Westminster Hospital, perhaps this is not so surprising.

4 'Treat your good nurses well'

1 The Factories and Workshops Acts of 1871, 1874, 1883 and 1891 introduced a range of measures to protect child workers, by lowering the maximum hours permitted and raising the minimum age. They also extended limited protection to adult workers. In 1871, the Trades Unions Act legalized such organizations, and in 1886, the Shop Hours Regulation Act made some attempt to control shop assistants' hours (Warren 2000).

2 The aim of the Early Closing Movement (which was the subject of the article) was to reduce hours of business generally, as the Factories Bill had done for factory workers.

3 An article in *The Times* illustrates the interchangeable use of the two terms: speakers at an 'Anti-sweating' demonstration in Hyde Park referred to 'the horrors of white slavery revealed by the inquiry of the Committee of the House of Lords' (*The Times*, 23 July 1888).

4 Morris was quoting figures from R. Mudie-Smith's *Sweated Industries: being a Handbook of the 'Daily News' Exhibition* (1906). Other sources have cited even lower wages for women in this sector. The Statistical Society put needlewomen's wages in St George's in the East at 5s 9d per week in 1860; while witnesses to 1890 Commission on Sweating reported shirtmakers earning just 1s 3d a week (G.S. Jones 1971: 109, 125).

5 Morris' figures for subsistence wages come from Cabdury and Shann's *Sweating* (1907). Edward Cadbury (1873–1948), son of George Cadbury, founder of the Bourneville chocolate company, 'had a passion for social reform [and] a parallel interest in education', according to his obituary in *The Times*. He was particularly interested in women's work and wages. He was also chairman of the *Daily News*, where he was responsible for that paper's liberal and progressive policy (*The Times*, 22 November 1948: 7).

6 This value of a nurse's board and lodging has been derived from several sources. Cadbury and Shann's upper limit of 16 shillings a week for a subsistence wage is equivalent to just over £40 a year. A retired nurse, in a letter to the *Nursing Record*, detailed her annual budget as follows: rent, gas, rates, taxes for a small house, £14; food, £26; coal and wood, £8; wine, £2.16s; clothing £4; incidental maintenance costs (e.g. chimney-sweep), £2. The total comes to £56 16s (Cadbury and Shann quoted in Morris 1986: 96; *NR*, 20 January 1894: 55). The figure of 19 shillings a week is the halfway point between these two.

7 Nurses' wages were similar at all the major London hospitals. In the provinces they may have been lower, although evidence from Birmingham General

Hospital suggests that by the end of the century any differential between the metropolis and the provinces was marginal (Wildman 1999).

8 The use of 'specials' (temporary nurses hired to deal with special cases or general staff shortages) and the problems associated with them is discussed in detail in Chapter 2.

9 This level of turnover may seem insupportable, but in 2002, a *BMJ* article claimed that inner London hospitals experienced similar attrition rates. It concluded: 'Turnover rates of more than one third are disruptive for staff and patients, as well as being costly' (Finlayson *et al.* 2002). A government report in 2007 found that London-based hospital trusts regarded even 10.5 per cent turnover in nurses to be a significant problem (Office of Manpower Economics 2008).

10 The increasing reliance on probationers at most hospitals has been discussed in Chapter 2. See Appendix 2 for a comparison of nursing departments in leading London hospitals in the early 1890s.

11 The length of notice was probably one month, judging by the example of Night Superintendent Jane Hope. She was asked to leave immediately, after being accused of several misdemeanours, but was given one month's pay in lieu of notice (SGHCON/1 8 October 1883).

12 Clara Jones was described in the minutes as the preferred candidate, but received no votes when the Committee gathered to ratify her appointment. The reason for their change of heart was not recorded (SGHCON/1, 20 December 1869; SGHCON/1, 3 January 1870). Only months after being turned down by St George's, she was appointed Matron at the Homerton Fever Hospital (1871 decennial census).

13 Mrs Dickin, the new Superintendent, brought eight years' experience from Liverpool Children's Hospital, and the prospect of working with a such an experienced woman might have given the HSC's voluntary, frankly amateur, sisters cause for concern.

14 At King's College Hospital a long dispute between the sisters of St John's House (who nursed the hospital), the hospital's managers and the Council of St John's House ended with the resignation of the Lady Superior. Many of the sisters left with her, leaving the managers of St John's House and King's to pick up the pieces (Moore 1988; Helmstadter 1993b; Jordan 1999).

15 Gregory's father was a Shropshire-based gentleman-farmer (SGHNDB).

16 In *The Hospital* writers fell into one of two camps: those who agreed with 'Doctor's Daughter', who was glad that some matrons would employ only 'gentlewomen as nurses' (*H/NM*, 13 September 1898); or those who agreed with another writer, who argued that lady nurses were stealing the 'bread from [those] who have no resource but to work for a living' (*H/NM*, 8 June 1889: xxxviii). The argument recurred throughout the 1890s, clearly illustrating the tensions which existed.

17 The numbers available for analysis (11 in total) are very small, so any conclusions can only be considered suggestive of a trend, rather than confirming it.

18 The optimum age is arrived at by assuming a three-year training period starting at age 25, a year as a ward nurse and then five years as a head nurse.

19 Several lady superintendents at the HSC survived only a few years. Miss Hicks, who had been 31 years old on appointment, resigned after only two years, being 'physically unfitted to continue'; while Miss Close, her successor (also 31) lasted four years before resigning through 'ill health' (GOS/1/2/17, 17 September 1890; GOS/1/2/20, 17 January 1894).

20 By comparison, Ethel Fenwick's successor, Isla Stewart, was 31 when she took up the role at Bart's in 1887 (McGann 1992).

21 See p. 108 for a pen portrait of Ann Moseley.

22 Mary Roberts went on to become Matron of the Queens Hospital in Birmingham, and returned to St George's in 1893 as Matron's Assistant.

23 The perilous nature of the hospital's finances was exposed at a public meeting in June 1869, when it was reported that it was necessary to 'eat into' the Hospital's reserves simply to keep going (SGHWB/35, 9 June 1869). For discussion of the financing of voluntary hospitals in the nineteenth century see Waddington 1996 and 2000.

24 These adverse changes, which hit head nurses hardest, had been introduced by Miss Veitch. Perhaps the root of subsequent problems between head nurses and Veitch's successor, Maria Gregory, can be found in these initiatives.

25 For examples of the arguments in favour of lady nurses, see *NR*, 10 October 1896; *H/NM*, 1 October 1898, 11 February 1899. Arguments against lady nurses, including that of stealing livelihoods from those who needed to work, can be found in *NR*, 10 January 1888; *H/NM*, 8 June 1889, 6 September 1890, 28 January 1899, 8 June 1899.

26 Examples of community spirit among nurses abound in the letters of the *Nursing Record* and *The Hospital*, particularly those asking colleagues to help nurses fallen on hard times. In one case, a retired matron had been rendered almost destitute through no fault of her own. Fellow nurses were asked to assist by contributing to a fund to help her back on her feet (*H/NM*, 30 June 1894). Several months later, Mrs Mortimer wrote to thank everyone who had contributed; the fund had enabled her to pay off her debts, restock her shop and set up a contingency against future disasters (*H/NM*, 29 September 1894). This case was not unusual.

27 The annual rise was withheld if a nurse's conduct was unsatisfactory. Head Nurse Jane Atkinson was found guilty of intoxication, and although retaining her position (on account of her 'long and efficient' service), her annual pay rise of £1 a year was suspended (SGHWB/33, 28 December 1864). Annual rises were common practice amongst London hospitals, so, as in other initiatives, St George's was not innovatory in this but merely trying to keep pace with competitors. In fact, the phenomenon of annual pay rises was common in many forms of employment. According to Frank Scudamore, an early proponent of women clerks in the Post Office, there was an expectation among workers generally that wages would rise each year, long after their contribution to the organization had peaked (Jordan 1996).

28 See Appendix 2 for a comparison of numbers of applicants to different London hospitals in the 1890s.

29 The reluctance to permit nurses to have fires, or to install gas lighting, was founded in a fear of fires breaking out, as much as the cost of such facilities. As late as 1894, the General Purpose Committee (responsible for the fabric of the building) rejected a proposal to install gas lighting in the nurses' accommodation, probably on the grounds of fire risk (SGHWB/57, 21 Nov 1894).

30 Grogan's book is discussed in more detail in Chapter 5.

31 A similar argument has been for shop work, which had an 'aura of middle class respectability [which] to many young people of the working classes ... represented a definite step upward in the social scale' (Holcombe 1973).

32 A special committee on the causes of dissatisfaction among nurses used this phrase to describe what needed to be done to induce nurses to remain at the hospital (SGHWB/33, 27 April 1864).

33 The Polytechnic at Regent Street (a forerunner of the University of Westminster) offered educational and training courses to the working population of London (of both sexes). Its Touring Association organized escorted tours to Europe. For a brief history of the early days of the Polytechnic see http://beginnings.ioe.ac.uk/begswest.html (accessed 22 August 2009). The National

Home Reading Union (dedicated to promoting the 'right sort' of reading among the working classes) offered walking holidays, which combined healthy recreation during the day with uplifting evening lecture programmes (Snape 2002).

34 Katherine Philippa Hicks (*c*.1857–?) daughter of a vicar, trained as a nurse at the Nightingale School. She was Night Superintendent at King's, before leading the Princess of Wales nurses in the Egyptian Campaign in 1885. On her return she was appointed Lady Superintendent at the HSC. She resigned in 1890, but was persuaded out of retirement to become head of the newly opened Nurses' Cooperation. She was outspoken and disapproving of nurse registration. In 1899, having resigned from the Cooperation, she married Mr Robert Emmott Large, a retired solicitor (*H/NM*, 27 April 1895; 'A Chat with Miss Hicks', *St James Gazette*, 29 November 1892; *H/NM*, 3 June 1899).

35 £15 was equivalent to at least 60 per cent of a St George's staff nurse's annual wages and 38 per cent of a sister's. Additionally, neither was entitled to one month's leave in a single year.

36 Fixed-term contracts implied an exchange of some sort, beyond the exchange of labour for wages. Probationers promised to remain for a predetermined period in return for their training and a certificate. In this scheme, new staff nurses signed a new fixed-term contract in return for extended leave. The hospital had found another tradable commodity.

37 Two-hour breaks, which had to be scheduled between meal breaks, doctors' rounds and visiting times, made organizing work rosters almost impossible. To accommodate the new off-duty hours, doctors were ordered to adhere 'strictly' to their ward round times, and changes were made to visiting times (SGHCON/2, 7 May 1894).

38 One nurse, writing about her experience, was particularly impressed by the refreshments: 'Everything was of the best, and unstinted in quantity; and the Nurses, fresh from the dull monotony of Hospital fare, evidently enjoyed the luxuries' (*NR*, 13 December 1888: 532).

39 Cycling was a controversial pastime for women, claimed by some to cause serious damage to a woman's reproductive system. Others held that, *in extremis*, it could lead to prostitution (Hargreaves 2001).

40 This is a common refrain among nurses, that tasks once considered an integral part of a nurse's job are eventually seen as detracting from it. In 2008, the Royal College of Nursing initiated a campaign for more administrative support for nurses, after a survey found that nurses spend 'a million hours a week on paperwork' (RCN 2009).

41 Medical officers formed close working relationships with their head nurses. One of the objectives of Nightingale's reforms had been to break this bond, transferring authority over nurses to the Matron (Baly 1987). Although St George's had been considered at the forefront of this movement with the appointment of Miss Veitch, in 1869, the reaction of the medical men to these changes suggest the hospital had slipped back into its old ways.

42 The deliberate construction of a career path, offering prospects of promotion, sets nursing apart from most other female occupations in the late nineteenth century, with the possible exception of teaching. Most employers went to great lengths to restrict women's access to promotion, by establishing separate women's departments and roles, which by definition did not lead to more senior positions. These were held precious for male employees (Anderson 1988). It is the investment in their training which encouraged hospitals to see their nurses as valuable assets, rather than disposable workers.

43 As Smedley had been the beneficiary of internal promotion herself (being promoted to sister at Bart's) it seems more likely that her abandonment of the

policy at St George's was linked to a lack of confidence in its nurses rather than disagreement with the practice.

44 Probationer Fowler, who joined in April 1893, was still in the hospital in November 1896, despite having completed her contract five months earlier. She was asked, politely, to resign. The manner of the request suggested that she had somehow managed to retain her post through oversight (SGHCON/2, 9 November 1896).

45 Four of these women came from hospitals Smedley knew well – three from Bart's and one from the HSC – illustrating the importance of networks for career advancement in Victorian nursing.

5 The development of nursing as a career

1 Attitudes to training women have been discussed in Chapter 3, and this view, that nursing was merely an interlude before marriage was echoed in arguments against all forms of training for women (Burman 1979).

2 Evidence from the nursing press is used here with caution, as correspondents were often anonymous, and influenced by political agendas. The politics of the two main nursing journals, the *Nursing Record* and *The Hospital*, are discussed in the Introduction and are easily discernible. If read with that knowledge, they offer a rare opportunity to hear the voice of ordinary nurses, albeit through the filter of editorial policy. Nursing was also the subject of articles and correspondence in other publications, such as *The Lady* and *Queen*, and newspapers such as *The Standard*, *The Times*, and the *Pall Mall Gazette*.

3 The segregation of female workers in the civil service and various other institutions is discussed in more detail in Chapter 1.

4 It was accepted that training to be a nurse equipped a woman with the necessary skills to be a successful wife and good mother (A. Crowther 2002).

5 This letter generated many responses, accusing the writer of adopting double standards and asking if the two men had been doctors, would she forbid her son from entering medical school? (*NR*, 7 July 1894).

6 Honnor Morten's, 'The Story of a Nurse', published in *The Graphic* (summer 1892: 14–22), and 'The Story of Miss O' (*H/NM*, 18 December 1886) are examples of the romanticized portrayal of nurses in women's journals.

7 Henry Burdett and Catherine Wood had an acrimonious relationship which became worse when she joined with Ethel Fenwick to set up the British Nursing Association in December 1887, in direct competition with the Hospital Association's own Sub-Committee of Nursing.

8 Burdett's argument that nursing was just one more way to earn a living was entirely contrary to Catherine Wood's view of nursing as a vocation, taken up as a moral duty and religious obligation.

9 The hospital's initiatives to counter this are discussed in detail in Chapter 4.

10 The data in Figure 5.1 were derived from Hospital Minute Books and Nurse Registers. Before 1866, the only source of information was the Weekly Board. Nurses who left appeared before it and the interview was minuted. The procedure was followed fitfully and evidence suggests that this source is not comprehensive. With the formation of the Committee of Nursing (in 1866) and the introduction of the Nurse Registers (in 1869), recording of movements in the Nursing Department became more formalized. Combined, these sources produce an arguably accurate representation of movements within the hospital's Nursing Department.

11 Given the seriousness with which the hospital treated dismissals, where no reason was recorded for a departure, it is assumed that such nurses left by choice. They have therefore been included in the totals for resignation.

12 Other employers took a very different view of marriage. Ellen Jordan has suggested that the inevitability of marriage generated a natural turnover in staff, which helped to suppress women's wages and reduced discontent at lack of promotion opportunities (Jordan 1999: 13). The argument was used to great effect in the Post Office, where Frank Scudamore successfully championed the employment of women as clerks, while allaying fears that they would threaten male jobs (Jordan 1996). Jordan has argued that hospital managers took a similar view, but evidence from the journals (and from this study) indicates that nursing was different. The heavy investment hospitals made in training nurses (unlike office or factory workers) made their loss – just as they were becoming skilled – both inefficient and disruptive.

13 The dip in resignations between 1873 and 1876 is hard to explain, but could be a reaction to the high number of leavers in 1872.

14 The groupings were developed for the study, the terms themselves were used in the Committee of Nursing or Weekly Board minute books to describe nurses' behaviour.

15 Until the latter part of the century, the domestic servants did not live in the hospital, so the relationship between them and the hospital's management would have been of a different nature.

16 Somerville also used the chaperone system. The system must have been rigidly enforced; there are records of complaints that at some lectures the chaperones took all the seats and students had to stand (Adams 1996: 33).

17 For further discussion of Victorian attitudes to relationships between the sexes, see Peterson 1989; Poovey 1989; Newton *et al.* 1983.

18 Ada Wilcockson (of the right age and place of birth) was found in the 1901 census living as a boarder in the house of a dental surgeon in Brighton. Her occupation was professional sick nurse. It seems likely that this is the same woman sacked from St George's for misconduct, and her career may not have been adversely affected by her dalliance.

19 *Enceinte* is French for pregnant. Its use here is typical of the Victorians' desire to couch unpleasant subjects in esoteric terms: another example is the use of Greek letters in medical notes to connote syphilis or tuberculosis.

20 In Victorian ideology, women were pure, innocent and asexual, but had within them the propensity to be sexual beings if they became tainted by sexual knowledge. The surveillance and control of young women's lives was designed to protect them from this knowledge. A pregnant single woman's condition was proof that she had fallen, succumbing to sexual desires, her reputation in tatters (Davidoff 1983).

21 The 1830 Beer Act reduced the price of beer to encourage drinkers to switch from gin and other spirits. Gin was believed to have a 'dangerously stimulating effect' on consumers; and the combination of gin and the working classes struck fear of uprising into the upper classes. Beer on the other hand was described as a 'moral species of beverage' (Harrison 1994: 70). The hospital's reasons for providing beer could have its roots in this earlier debate.

22 The death rate was calculated by taking the average number of deaths per year, and expressing this as a percentage of the average number of nurses on staff during the period. The most frequent causes of death were infectious fevers, including typhoid (over 30 per cent) and diphtheria, influenza and smallpox (20 per cent).

23 Nursing became one of the *Pall Mall Gazette's* campaigns. It was particularly critical of the London, sending in 'a special correspondent' under cover as a new probationer. The resulting report was damning of nurses' treatment, and singled out the Matron (Eva Luckes) for particular criticism, stating, '[She]

never comes into the wards ... she doesn't like the look of sick people, evidently' (*Pall Mall Gazette*, 18 July 1893, 19 July 1893).

24 Six probationers died, four from infectious fevers.

25 According to Fenwick, probationers were most susceptible during the first six months while acclimatizing to the hospital environment. She advocated more time off for probationers, who traditionally had the least amount of leave among all nurses, and shortening their working day to ten hours (Fenwick 1893). Her evidence on probationers' health is supported by the findings at St George's, but before any broad conclusions can be reached more detailed work is needed on other hospitals. The occupational health of nurses in the period 1890 to 1919 is the focus of doctoral research by Deborah Palmer at the University of Exeter.

26 James Riley's method for calculating prevalence was used: the total number of days lost to sickness in a year, divided by the total number of nurses on staff (Riley 1997).

27 James Riley's study on the Ancient Order of Foresters, a friendly society which covered the whole of Britain, included annual statistics on sickness among its members, who represented a diverse range of occupations and trades.

28 This is a curious finding, as Riley says in his introduction to the section that women were more likely to be sick than men. His data do not bear this out, but he does not discuss this apparent anomaly in his results.

29 Riley's study of customs agents in London in 1857–74 showed that while phthisis (respiratory tuberculosis) accounted for 31 per cent of deaths among this group, it only caused 1.4 per cent of sicknesses and 8 per cent of sickness time (Riley 1997: 195).

30 Back injuries are the plague of nurses in modern times. According to an article in the *Daily Telegraph* in 1996, back injuries to nurses were costing the National Health Service £1 million a week in lost working hours (Hall 1996).

31 The reappearance of the category in 1893 reflected the decision of seven probationers to leave within their initial two-month probationary period, presumably having decided nursing was not for them. SGHWB/56, 28 April 1894.

32 The committee was obviously annoyed by this incident, through which they lost a valuable nurse. The surgeon was severely reprimanded by the Medical School Committee and warned that he would be asked to resign if he behaved in a similar way again.

33 The increasing acceptance of nursing as a suitable occupation for daughters of respectable families may be linked to the perceived benefit of having a trained nurse in the family. This would prove very useful in times of sickness, and could also offer savings to the family economy.

34 Susan Crandle was not unique in being a hospital nurse and the mother of small children. St George's attitude to employing mothers as nurses has been discussed in Chapter 2.

35 Stanley's friends also advised her that she should leave. The role of 'friends' in a woman's decision to become a nurse or to leave suggests a close support network for many women, which was maintained even when they had ostensibly withdrawn from the outside world. Two other nurses gave 'friends' advice' as their reason for leaving the hospital.

36 One of the primary functions of the Nurse Register was to aid the Matron in drawing up the very valuable references for any nurses who left. These documents were essential for the continuation of a successful nursing career.

37 'Women and their Work' was a regular feature in the *Nursing Record*. The first column appeared on 31 October 1889.

38 Census figures for nursing can be misleading. The term was used very loosely, and was not restricted to trained professional nurses. However, while actual numbers may be exaggerated the general trends can probably be relied upon.

39 This value of a nurse's board and lodging is discussed in Chapter 4.
40 Harriett Kendall, night superintendent at St George's, finished her career as head of a nursing home in Torquay. See Pen Portrait 4, Harriett Kendall, p. 140, for a biography of this nurse.
41 For a brief biography of Philippa Hicks see Chapter 4, note 34.
42 Private nursing institutes proliferated in the late century, as can be seen from the advertising pages of the *Nursing Record*. There was no control or regulation over these agencies and the growing demand for private nurses created good opportunities for the financially astute. Many founders of nursing institutions were accused of greed and having no philanthropic motives for their businesses (Abel-Smith 1960: 58).
43 Even those who paid their nurses a percentage of actual earnings, rather than a flat wage, generally underpaid their staff; the worst were reported to be taking between 25 per cent and 40 per cent of a nurse's total earnings, in commission (Abel-Smith 1960: 58).
44 The formation of the Cooperation was reported in *The Hospital* as an initiative of a group of private nurses, although Henry Burdett was certainly involved from the earliest days and was a member of the original committee (Abel-Smith 1960: 59; *H/NM*, 24 January 1891: lxxxix; *NR*, 20 December 1902: 514).
45 It was so successful that there were calls in the press from disappointed nurses for more institutions to operate on the same, not-for-profit basis (*H/NM*, 12 November 1892).
46 If Burdett was a major backer of the project, there are contradictions at play which are difficult to explain. He was a strong supporter of hospital management and the supremacy of the voluntary sector, yet appeared to back independence for this group of nurses. Ethel Fenwick, who supported autonomy for nurses within the hospital sector, argued strenuously against independent private nursing institutions, maintaining they should always be associated with hospitals. As usual, the traditional enemies lined up against each other. The *Nursing Record* published many attacks on Burdett's involvement with the Nurses' Cooperation, claiming that financial gain was his main motivation.
47 If board and lodging was worth £50, a hospital nurse needed to earn £90 to match the private nurse's salary.
48 The heroine of Henry James' story had her own plan for social elevation, being determined to remain in her job as a telegraph operator in Mayfair, where she came into daily contact with the upper classes, rather than move to the suburbs with her less well-placed fiancé.
49 In addition to the Strangers' Hospital at Rio, there were hospitals at São Paulo (Hospital Samaritano) and Buenos Aires (the British Hospital) (*NR*, 18 January 1902: 49).
50 The enhanced mobility of female teacher trainers compared to their male counterparts can probably be explained by the lack of family responsibilities. It could be argued that this superior mobility of single women could confer advantage in a competitive job market.
51 Robinson's teachers, like the St George's nurses, were also prepared to move abroad, to outposts of the colonies, in pursuit of new challenges.
52 Alice Raynes and Ellen Parham may have been examples of hospital trained nurses encouraged to move into the workhouse system in order to improve the quality of nursing there (White 1978; Maggs 1983; Kirby 2002).

References

Primary sources: unpublished archives

St George's Hospital

The St George's Hospital Archive was held at the library of St George's Medical School, but has since relocated to the London Metropolitan Archive. The archive had not been comprehensively catalogued. The following abbreviations are used throughout this study to denote individual items within the collection:

SGHAR   St George's Hospital Annual Reports
SGHWB   St George's Hospital Weekly Board Minutes 1836–1900 (volumes 24–61)
SGHCON   St George's Hospital Committee of Nursing Minutes 1868–1900 (volumes 1–2)
SGHNR   St George's Hospital Nurse Registers 1870–1900 (volumes 1–6)
SGHRO   St George's Hospital Rules and Orders (eighteenth century)
SGHGPC   St George's Hospital General Purpose Committee, 1878–1900
SGHMC   St George's Hospital Medical School Committee, 1871–87
SGHNDB   The database created of nursing records from the St George's Archive, the census returns and other sources (See Apendix 1 for details)

The Charles Booth Archive

The archive is housed at the London School of Economics and Political Sciences. It is fully catalogued, and the catalogue is searchable online at http://booth.lse.ac.uk/. Items relevant to this study:

Booth A27   Collection of completed questionnaires from London hospitals regarding their nursing departments (1896)

Booth B153   Collection of interviews with matrons of London hospitals
and 154   (1896)

The interviews have been referenced by the Booth Collection Catalogue
reference, surname of the interviewee and date of interview.

The Hospital for Sick Children at Great Ormond Street (HSC)

The archive is housed within the Great Ormond Street Hospital for
Children, in London. It is extensively catalogued. The following items
were consulted for this study:

GOS/1/2/1–21   HSC Committee of Management Minutes (CM)
   1850–1900
GOS/11/1/10   Dr Charles West, Letter to the Chairman and Managing
   Committee of the Hospital for Sick Children, 20
   January 1876
GOS/5/2/30–31   Lady Superintendent's Report Book, 1860–81
GOS/5/2/49   Rules for Nurses (1897)
GOS/5/2/1   Register of Sisters and Staff Nurses

Manchester Royal Infirmary (MRI)

The archive for the MRI is held at the hospital. It is uncatalogued.

MRIWB   Manchester Royal Infirmary Weekly Board Minutes, October
   1864.

Primary sources: published

Official documents

*Report from the Select Committee of the House of Lords on Metropolitan Hospitals, together
with the Proceedings of the Committee, Minutes, Evidence and Appendix* (HoLSC/MH)
London: Eyre & Spottiswoode, 1890.
Third Report from the House of Lords Select Committee on Metropolitan Hospitals (HoLSC/
MH3) London: Eyre & Spottiswoode, 1892.
1st to 5th Report from the House of Lords Committee on the Sweating System, 1888–90.
(HoLSC/SS)

Newspapers and journals

British Medical Journal (BMJ)
The Daily News
The Graphic
The Lady

The Lancet
The Pall Mall Gazette
The Queen
St George's Medical Gazette
The St James Gazette
The Times

Nursing journals

Nursing Notes
The Nursing Record (1888–92)/*Nursing Record and Hospital World* (1893–1902)/*The British Journal of Nursing* (1903) (*NR*)
The Hospital (Nursing Mirror Supplement) (1886–1900) (*H/NM*)

Secondary sources

Abbott, A. (1988) *The System of Professions: an essay on the division of expert labour*, Chicago: University of Chicago Press.
Abel-Smith, B. (1960) *A History of the Nursing Profession*, London: Heinemann.
Abel-Smith, B. (1964) *The Hospitals, 1800–1948: a study in social administration in England and Wales*, London: Heinemann.
Adams, P. (1996) *Somerville for Women: an Oxford college, 1879–1993*, Oxford: Oxford University Press.
Alexander, S. (1976) 'Women's Work in Nineteenth-Century London', in J. Mitchell and A. Oakley (eds) *The Rights and Wrongs of Women*, London: Penguin, pp. 59–111.
Alexandra Hospital for Children with Hip Disease (2007) Biographical History. Online. Available at www.aim25.ac.uk (accessed on 2 January 2009).
Allen, D. (2001) *The Changing Shape of Nursing Practice: the role of nurses in the hospital division of labour*, London: Routledge.
Anderson, G. (1988) *The White Blouse Revolution*, Manchester: Manchester University Press.
Anon. (1887) 'Private Nursing', *The Hospital*, 26 February.
Anon. (1891) 'Nursing as a Profession for Women', *The Nursing Record*, 29 January, p. 53.
Armstrong, W.A. (1972) 'The Use of Information about Occupation', in E.A. Wrigley (ed.) *Essays in the Use of Quantitative Methods for the Study of Social Data*, Cambridge: Cambridge University Press, pp. 191–225.
Ayers, G.M. (1971) *England's First State Hospitals and the Metropolitan Asylums Board*, London: Wellcome Institute for the History of Medicine.
Baly, M. (1986 [1997]) *Florence Nightingale and the Nursing Legacy* (2nd edition), London: Whurr.
Baly, M. (1987) 'Nightingale Nurses', in C. Maggs (ed.) *Nursing History: the state of the art*, London, Croom Helm, pp. 33–59.
Barker, G.F.R. (2004) 'Denison (John) Evelyn, Viscount Ossington (1800–1873)', *Oxford Dictionary of National Biography*, Oxford: Oxford University Press. Online. Available at www.oxforddnb.com (accessed on 23 August 2006).
Bashford, A. (1998) *Purity and Pollution: gender, embodiment and Victorian medicine*, Basingstoke: Macmillan.

Besant, A. (1888) 'What Can the Match Girls Do?' *Pall Mall Gazette*, 9 July.

Best, G. (1979 [1985]) *Mid-Victorian Britain, 1851–1875*, London: Fontana.

Blake, C. (1990) *The Charge of the Parasols*, London: The Women's Press.

Blomfield, J. (1933) *St George's, 1733–1933*, London: Medici Society.

Boase, G.C. (2004) 'Bouverie, Edward Pleydell (1818–1889)', *Oxford Dictionary of National Biography*, Oxford: Oxford University Press. Online. Available at www.oxforddnb.com (accessed on 23 August 2006).

Borsay, A. (2006) 'Nursing History: an irrelevance for practice?' Paper delivered at the Third Annual History of Nursing Conference: Race Class and Gender: the evolution of the modern nursing culture, 14 November 2006, London.

Boyd, H. (1991) *The Age of Atonement: the influence of Evangelicalism on social and economic thought, 1875–1865*, Oxford: Clarendon Press.

Bradshaw, A. (2000) *The Nurse Apprentice, 1860–1977*, Aldershot: Ashgate.

Brooks, J. (2001) 'Structured by Class, Bound by Gender: nursing and special probationer schemes, 1860–1939', *International History of Nursing Journal* 6 (2), pp. 13–21.

Brooks, J. and Rafferty, A.M. (2007) 'Dress and Distinction in Nursing, 1860–1939: "A corporate (as well as corporeal) armour of probity and purity"', *Women's History Review* 16 (1), pp. 41–57.

Burdett, H. (1890) 'Nurses' Food, Work and Hours of Recreation', *The Hospital (Nursing Mirror Supplement)*, 29 November, pp. 135–7.

Burdett, H. (1900) *Burdett's Hospitals and Charities 1900*. Online. Available at www.victorianlondon.org/health/dickens-hospitals.htm (accessed on 24 April 2009).

Burman, S. (1979) 'Introduction', in S. Burman (ed.) *Fit Work for Women*, London: Croom Helm, pp. 9–14.

Burstyn, J. (1980) *Victorian Education and the Ideal of Womanhood*, London: Croom Helm.

Bynum, W. (2001) 'Hospitalism', *The Lancet* 357, p. 1372.

Cannadine, D. (1998) *Class in Britain*, New Haven, CT: Yale University Press.

Carpenter, M. (1980) 'Asylum Nursing before 1914: a chapter in the history of labour', in C. Davies (ed.) *Rewriting Nursing History*, London: Routledge, pp. 123–46.

Clark-Kennedy, A.E. (1962–3) *The London: a study in the voluntary hospital system*, London: Pitman Medical.

Collins, S. and Parker, E. (2003) 'Eva Luckes: a Victorian matron', *International History of Nursing Journal* 7 (3), pp. 66–74.

Cominos, P. (1980) 'Innocent *Femina Sensualis*', in M. Vicinus (ed.) *Suffer and Be Still: women in the Victorian age*, London: Methuen, pp. 155–72.

Community of St Peter, Kilburn, Woking and elsewhere (n.d.) Records 1861–2004, reference number 7805. Online. Available at www.exploringsurreyspast.org.uk/GetRecord/SHCOL_7805 (accessed 2 May 2009).

Cordery, S. (1995) 'Friendly Societies and the Discourse of Respectability in Britain, 1825–1875', *Journal of British Studies* 34, pp. 35–58.

Corfield, P. (1995) *Power and the Professions, 1700–1850*, London: Routledge.

Crowther, A. (2002) 'Why Women Should Be Nurses and not Doctors', UK Centre for History of Nursing Seminar Papers 2000–1. Online. Available at www.nursing.manchester.ac.uk/ukchnm/publications/seminarpapers (accessed 27 September 2009).

Crowther, M.A. (1981) *The Workhouse System, 1834–1929: the history of an English social institution*, Athens, GA: University of Georgia Press.

D'Antonio, P. (1999) 'Revisiting and Rethinking the Rewriting of History', *Bulletin of the History of Medicine* 73, pp. 269–90.

D'Cruze, S. (2000) 'On Women and the Family', in June Purvis (ed.) *Women's History: Britain, 1850–1945*, London: Routledge, pp. 51–82.

Damant, M. (2005) 'District Nursing: professional skills and knowledge in domestic settings: linking national and local networks of expertise, 1866–1974', unpublished thesis, University of Leicester.

Darley, G. (2006), 'Octavia Hill (1838–1912)', *Oxford Dictionary of National Biography*, Oxford: Oxford University Press. Online. Available at www.oxforddnb.com/view/article/33873 (accessed 14 December 2006).

Davidoff, L. (1983) 'Class and Gender in Victorian England', in J. Newton, M. Ryan and J. Walkowitz (eds) *Sex and Class in Women's History*, London: Routledge and Kegan Paul, pp. 16–71.

Davidoff, L. and Hall, C. (2002) *Family Fortunes: men and women of the English middle class* (revised edition), London: Routledge.

Davies, C. (1980) 'Introduction', in C. Davies (ed.) *Rewriting Nursing History*, London: Croom Helm, pp. 11–17.

Davies, C. (2007) 'Rewriting Nursing History – Again', *Nursing History Review* 15, pp. 11–28.

Davin, A. (2005) 'City Girls: young women, new employment and the city, London 1880–1910', in M. Maynes, B. Soland and C. Benninghaus (eds) *Secret Gardens, Satanic Mills: placing girls in European history, 1750–1960*, Bloomington, IN: Indiana University Press, pp. 209–23.

Dean, M. and Bolton, G. (1980) 'The Administration of Poverty and the Development of Nursing Practice in Nineteenth-Century England', in C. Davies (ed.) *Rewriting Nursing History*, London: Croom Helm, pp. 76–101.

Deane, T. (1996) 'Late Nineteenth-Century Philanthropy: the case for Louisa Twining', in A. Digby and J. Stewart (eds) *Gender, Health and Welfare*, London: Routledge, pp. 122–42.

Dent, C. (1894a) 'A History of Nursing at St George's I', *St George's Hospital Gazette* II (13), pp. 41–9.

Dent, C. (1894b) 'A History of Nursing at St George's II', *St George's Hospital Gazette* II (14), pp. 61–71.

Dent, C. (1894c) 'A History of Nursing at St George's III', *St George's Hospital Gazette* II (15), pp. 82–9.

Dent, C. (1894d) 'Lectures at St George's Hospital', *The Hospital (Nursing Mirror Supplement)*, 3 March, p. ccxv.

Digby, A. (1992) 'Victorian Values and Women', in T. Smout (ed.) *Victorian Values*, Oxford: Oxford University Press, pp. 195–216.

Digby, A. and Stewart, J. (1996) 'Welfare in Context', in A. Digby and J. Stewart (eds) *Gender, Health and Welfare*, London: Routledge, pp. 1–31.

Dingwall, R., Rafferty, A.M. and Webster, C. (1988) *An Introduction to the Social History of Nursing*, London: Routledge.

Domville, E.J. (1888) *A Manual for Hospital Nurses and Others Engaged in Caring for the Sick*, London: J. and A. Churchill.

Duckworth, D. (1897) 'Introduction', in C. Weekshaw and W.A. Radford *A Text-Book of Nursing*, London: Edward Arnold, pp. vii–ix.

Dyhouse, C. (1976) 'Social Darwinistic Ideas and the Development of Women's Education in England', *History of Education* 5 (1), pp. 41–58.

Dyhouse, C. (1981) *Girls Growing up in Late Victorian and Edwardian England*, London: Routledge and Kegan Paul.

Erichsen, J. (1874) *On Hospitalism and the Causes of Death After Operations*, London.

Evans, R.J. (2000) *In Defence of History*, London: Granta.

Fenwick, E. (1889) 'The Overstrain of Nursing – 1', *The Nursing Record*, 21 October.

Fenwick, E. (1893) *Nursing Record and Hospital World*, 28 October.

Finlayson, B., Dixon, J., Meadows, S.and Blair, G., (2002) 'Mind the Gap: the extent of the NHS nursing shortage', *British Medical Journal*, 325 (7 September), pp 538–41.

Foucault, M. (trans A. Sheridan) (1991) *The Birth of the Clinic: an archaeology of medical perception*, London: Vintage.

Foucault, M. (trans A. Sheridan) (1994) *Discipline and Punish: the birth of the prison*, London: Penguin.

French, C. and Tilley, P. (1997) 'Record Linkage for Nineteenth Century Census Returns: automatic or computer aided?' *History and Computing* 9, pp. 122–33.

Gamarnikow, E. (1978) 'Women's Employment and the Sexual Division of Labour: the case for nursing', in A. Kuhn and A. Wolpe (eds) *Feminism and Materialism: women and modes of production*, London: Routledge and Kegan Paul, 1978, pp. 98–123.

Gamarnikow, E. (1991) 'Nurse or Woman: gender and professionalism in reformed nursing, 1860–1923', in P. Holden and J. Littleworth (eds) *Anthropology and Nursing*, London: Routledge, pp. 110–29.

Gleadle, K. (2001) *British Women in the Nineteenth Century*, Basingstoke: Palgrave Macmillan.

Godden, J. (2003) 'Matching the Idea? The first generation of Nightingale nursing probationers, Sydney Hospital, 1868–84', *Health and History* 5 (1), pp. 22–41.

Gould, T. and Uttley, D. (1997) *A Short History of St George's Hospital and the Origins of Its Ward Names*, London: Athlone Press.

Granshaw, L. (1981) 'St Thomas' Hospital, London, 1850–1900', unpublished thesis, Bryn Mawr College, Pennsylvania, USA.

Grogan, M. (1880) *How Women May Earn Their Living*, London: Cassell, Petter.

Group, T.M. and Roberts, J. (2001) *Nursing, Physician Control, and the Medical Monopoly: historical perspectives on gendered inequality in roles, rights, and range of practice*, Bloomington, IN: Indiana University Press.

Hall, C. (1979) 'The Early Formation of Victorian Domestic Ideology', in S. Burman (ed.) *Fit Work for Women*, London: Croom Helm, pp. 15–32.

Hall, C. (1996) 'Bill for Nurses' Back Injuries is £1 Million a Week', *Daily Telegraph*, 4 April, 1996. Online. Available at www.telegraph.co.uk (accessed on 19 January, 2007. Link now broken).

Hannam, J. (2004a) 'Paget, Dame (Mary) Rosalind (1855–1948)', *Oxford Dictionary of National Biography*, Oxford: Oxford University Press. Online. Available at www.oxforddnb.com (accessed 21 March 2005).

Hannam, J. (2004b) 'Smith, Zepharina Philadelphia (1836–1894)', *Oxford Dictionary of National Biography*, Oxford: Oxford University Press. Online. Available at www.oxforddnb.com (accessed 21 March 2005).

Hardy, A. (1994) 'Death Is the Cure: using the General Register Office cause of death statistics for 1837–1920', *Social History of Medicine* 7, pp. 472–92.

Hargreaves, J. (2001) 'The Victorian Cult of the Family and the Early Years of

Female Sport', in S. Scraton and A. Flintoff (eds) *Gender and Sport: a reader*, London: Routledge, pp. 53–65.

Harris, J. (1993) *Private Lives, Public Spirit: Britain, 1870–1914*, London: Penguin.

Harrison, B. (1994) *Drink and the Victorians: the temperance question in England, 1815–1872* (2nd edition), Keele: Keele University Press.

Hawkins, S. (2010) 'From Maid to Matron: nursing as a route to social advancement in nineteenth-century England', *Women's History Review* 19 (1), pp. 125–43.

Haywood, R.A. (1998) 'Changing Concept of Infection and Its Influence on Hospital Design', unpublished thesis, Keele University.

Helmstadter, C. (1993a) 'Old and New: nurses in London teaching hospitals', *Nursing History Review* 1, pp. 43–70.

Helmstadter, C. (1993b) 'Robert Bentley Todd, St Johns House and the Origins of the Modern Trained Nurse', *Bulletin of the History of Medicine* 67, pp. 282–319.

Helmstadter, C. (1994) 'Passing of the Nightwatch: night nursing reforms in London teaching hospitals, 1856–1890', *Canadian Bulletin of Medical History* 11 (1), pp. 23–69.

Helmstadter, C. (1996) 'Nurse Recruitment and Retention in Nineteenth-Century London Teaching Hospitals', *International History of Nursing Journal* 2 (1), pp. 58–69.

Helmstadter, C. (2001) 'From Private to Public Sphere: the first generation of lady nurses', *Nursing History Review* 9, pp. 127–40.

Helmstadter, C. (2002) 'Early Nursing Reform in Nineteenth-Century London: a doctor-driven phenomonen', *Medical History* 46 (3), pp. 325–50.

Helmstadter, C. (2003) 'A Real Tone: professionalising nursing', *Nursing History Review* 11, pp. 3–30.

Higgs, E. (1986) 'Domestic Service and Household Production', in A. John (ed.) *Unequal Opportunities: women's employment in England 1800–1918*, Oxford: Basil Blackwell, pp. 125–52.

Higgs, E. (2005) *Making Sense of the Census Revisited: census records for England and Wales 1801–1901*, London: Institute of Historical Research.

Holcombe, L. (1973) *Victorian Ladies at Work*, Newton Abbott: David and Charles.

Hollis, P. (1987) *Ladies Elect: women in English local government, 1865–1914*, Oxford: Clarendon Press.

Holmes, T. (1888) *The Hospital (Nursing Mirror Supplement)*, 18 February, p. 356.

Horn, P. (1999) *Pleasures and Pastimes in Victorian Britain*, Stroud: Sutton.

Hudson, P. (1999) 'Industrialisation in Britain: the challenge of micro-history', *Family and Community History* 2 (1), pp. 5–16.

Humphry, L. (1898) *A Manual of Nursing Medical and Surgical*, London: Charles Griffin.

James, H. (1898/2001) *In the Cage, Henry James Collected Tales*, London: Penguin Classics.

Jamieson, E.M., Sewall, M.F. and Suhrie, E.B. (1966) *Trends in Nursing History: their social, international and ethical relationships*, Philadelphia, PA: Saunders.

John, A. (1986) 'Introduction', in A. John (ed.) *Unequal Opportunities: women's employment in England 1800–1918*, Oxford: Basil Blackwell.

Johnson, R. (1970) 'Educational Policy and Social Control in Early Victorian England', *Past and Present* 49, pp. 96–119.

Jones, G.S. (1971) *Outcast London: a study in the relationship between classes in Victorian society*, Oxford: Clarendon Press.

Jones, K. (1972) *A History of the Mental Health Services*, London: Routledge and Kegan Paul.

Jordan, E. (1996) 'The Lady Clerks at the Prudential: the beginning of vertical segregation by sex in clerical work in nineteenth-century Britain', *Gender and History* 8, pp. 65–81.

Jordan, E. (1999) *The Women's Movement and Women's Employment in Nineteenth-Century Britain*, London: Routledge.

Jordan, E. (2002) ' "Suitable and Remunerative Employment": the feminization of hospital dispensing in late nineteenth-century England', *Social History of Medicine* 15 (3), pp. 429–56.

Judd, C. (1998) *Bedside Seductions: nursing and the Victorian imagination, 1830–1880*, Basingstoke: Macmillan.

King, S. (2006) *Women, Welfare and Local Politics, 1880–1902: 'we might be trusted'*, Brighton: Sussex Academic.

Kirby, S. (2002) 'Reciprocal Rewards: British Poor Law nursing and the campaign for state registration', *International History of Nursing Journal* 7 (2), pp. 4–13.

Lancaster, M.-J. (ed.) (2002) *Letters of Engagement, 1884–1888: the love letters of Adrian Hope and Laura Trowbridge*, London: Tite Street Press.

Langland, E. (1995) *Nobody's Angels: middle-class women and domestic ideology*, London: Cornell University Press.

Levine, P. (1990) *Feminist Lives in Victorian England: private roles and public commitment*, Oxford: Basil Blackwell.

Lewis, J. (1991) *Women and Social Action in Victorian and Edwardian Britain*, Aldershot: Edward Elgar.

Likeman, J. (2002) 'Nursing at UCH, 1862–1948', unpublished thesis, University College London.

Lumsden, K. (1896) 'Training in Children's Hospitals', *Nursing Record*, 21 March, 1896, p. 242.

Lynaugh, J. (2005) 'Common Working Ground', in B. Mortimer and S. McGann (eds) *New Directions in the History of Nursing: international perspectives*, London: Routledge, pp. 194–202.

McDermid, J. (1995). 'Women and Education', in J. Purvis (ed.) *Women's History: Britain, 1850–1945: an introduction*, London: UCL Press, pp. 107–30.

McGann, S. (1992) *Battle of the Nurses: a study of eight women who influenced the development of professional nursing, 1880–1930*, London: Scutari Press.

McGann, S. (2002) 'The Wind of Change is Blowing', *Nursing History Review* 10, pp. 21–32.

Maggs, C. (1980) 'Nurse Recruitment in Four Provincial Hospitals 1881–1921', in C. Davies (ed.) *Rewriting Nursing History*, London: Croom Helm, pp. 18–40.

Maggs, C. (1983) *The Origins of General Nursing*, London: Croom Helm.

Maggs, C. (1987) 'Profit and Loss and the Hospital Nurse', in C. Maggs (ed.) *Nursing History: the state of the art*, London: Croom Helm, pp. 176–89.

Mangion, C. (2008) *Contested Identities: Catholic women religious in nineteenth-century England and Wales*, Manchester: Manchester University Press.

Meehan, T.C. (2003) 'Careful Nursing: a model for contemporary nursing practice', *Journal of Advanced Nursing* 44 (1), pp. 99–107.

Miller, P. (2005) British Medical Association, 10 November 2005, quoted in 'Nurse Prescribing Plans Opposed', BBC News Online. Available at http://news.bbc.co.uk/1/hi/health/4424112.stm (accessed 26 June 2009).

Mills, D. (1999) 'The Trouble with Farms at the Census Office: an evaluation of farm statistics from the censuses of 1851–1881 in England and Wales', *Agricultural History Review*, 47, pp. 58–77.

Mills, D. and Schurer, K. (1996) 'Employment and Occupation', in D. Mills and K. Schurer (eds) *Local Communities and the Victorian Census Enumerator Books*, Oxford: Leopard's Head Press, pp. 136–60.

Moore, J. (1988) *A Zeal for Responsibility. the struggle for professional nursing in Victorian England, 1868–1883*, Athens, GA: University of Georgia Press.

Morris, J. (1986) 'The Characteristics of Sweating: the late nineteenth-century London and Leeds tailoring trade', in A. John (ed.) *Unequal Opportunities: women's employment in England, 1800–1918*, Oxford: Basil Blackwell, pp. 95–121.

Morten, H. (1892). *How to Become a Nurse and How to Succeed*, London: Scientific Press.

Mortimer, B. (2005) 'History of Nursing: past, present and future', in Barbara Mortimer and Susan McGann (eds) *New Directions in the History of Nursing: international perspectives*, London: Routledge, pp. 1–21.

Newton, J., Ryan, M. and Walkowitz, J. (1983) *Sex and Class in Women's History*, London: Routledge and Kegan Paul.

Nightingale, F. (1861 [1952]) *Notes on Nursing*, London: Gerald Duckworth.

Office of Manpower Economics (2008) 'Workforce Survey Results for Nursing Staff, Midwives and Health Visitors, 2007', London: Office of Manpower Economics. Online. Available at www.ome.uk.com/review.cfm?body=6 (accessed on 22 August 2009).

Parker, J. (1988) *Women and Welfare: ten Victorian women in public service*, London: Macmillan.

Parry, N. and Parry, J. (1976) *The Rise of the Medical Profession: a study of collective social mobility*, London: Croom Helm.

Pavey, A. (1938) *The Story of the Growth of Nursing as an Art, a Vocation, and a Profession*, London: Faber and Faber.

Pedersen, J. (2002) 'Enchanting Modernity: invention of tradition at two women's colleges', *History of Universities* 17, pp. 162–91.

Perkin, J. (1993) *Victorian Women*, London: John Murray.

Peterson, M.J. (1989) *Family, Love, and Work in the Lives of Victorian Gentlewomen*, Bloomington, IN: Indiana University Press.

Pinker, R. (1966) *English Hospital Statistics 1861–1938*, London: Heinemann.

Plarr, V. (1930) *Plarr's Lives of the Fellows of the Royal College of Surgeons: revised by Sir D'Arcy Power, W.G. Spencer and G.E. Gask*, London: Simpkin Marshall.

Poovey, M. (1989) *Uneven Developments: the ideological work of gender in mid-Victorian England*, London: Virago.

Postan, M.M. (1971) *Fact and Relevance: essays on historical method*, London: Cambridge University Press.

Prochaska, F. (1980). *Women and Philanthropy in Nineteenth-Century England*, Oxford: Clarendon Press.

Rafferty, A.M. (1995) 'The Anomaly of Autonomy: space and status in early nursing reform', *International History of Nursing Journal* 1 (1), pp. 43–56.

Rafferty, A.M. (1996) *The Politics of Nursing Knowledge*, London: Routledge.

Rafferty, A.M. and Solano, D. (2007) 'The Rise and Demise of the Colonial Nursing Service: British nurses in the colonies, 1896–1966', *Nursing History Review* 15, pp. 147–54.

RCN (Royal College of Nursing) (2009) 'Survey Shows Nurses Spend More Than a Million Hours a Week on Paperwork', 22 August 2009. Online. Available at www.rcn.org.uk/newsevents/news/article/uk/rcn_survey_shows_nurses_spend_more_than_a_million_hours_a_week_on_paperwork (accessed 22 August 2009).

Riley, J. (1997) *Sick not Dead: the health of British workingmen during the mortality decline*, Baltimore, MD: Johns Hopkins University Press.

Rivett, G. (1986) *The Development of the London Hospital System, 1823–1982*, London: King Edward's Hospital Fund for London.

Robinson W. (2000) 'Women and Teacher Training, 1880–1914', in J. Goodman and S. Harrop (eds) *Women, Educational Policy-making and Administration in England: authoritative women since 1800* (Routledge Research in Gender and History, 4), London: Routledge, pp. 99–115.

Rose, S.O. (1992) *Limited Livelihoods: gender and class in nineteenth-century England*, London: Routledge.

Ryle, J.C. (*c.*1870) 'The Teaching of the Ritualists not the Teaching of the Church of England', Church Association Tract 4. Online. Available at www.churchsociety.org/publications/catracts.htm (accessed 1 August 2009).

Simnet, A. (1986) 'The Pursuit of Respectability: women and the nursing profession, 1860–1900', in R. White (ed.) *Political Issues in Nursing: past, present and future*, vol. 2, Chichester: John Wiley and Sons, pp. 1–24.

Simonton, D. (2001) 'Nursing History as Women's History', *International History of Nursing Journal* 6 (1), pp. 35–47.

Smith, F.B. (1982) *Florence Nightingale: reputation and power*, London: Croom Helm.

Smith, F.B. (1995) 'The Russian Influenza in the United Kingdom, 1889–1894', *Social History of Medicine* 8 (1), pp. 55–73.

Snape, R. (2002) 'The National Home Reading Union, 1889–1930', *Journal of Victorian Culture* 7 (1), pp. 86–110.

Steele, Dr (1871) 'Report on the Nursing Arrangements of the London Hospitals', in C.H. Fagge (ed.) *Guy's Hospital Reports* 3 (XVI), pp. 540–55.

Steinbach, S. (2004) *Women in England, 1760–1914: a social history*, London: Phoenix.

Stephenson, M.V. (1940) *The First Fifty Years of the Training School for Nurses for the Hospital of the University of Pennsylvania*, Philadelphia, PA: J.B. Lippincott Company.

Stone, L. (1971) 'Prosopography', *Daedalus* 100, pp. 46–79.

Strachey, L. 1918 [2003] *Eminent Victorians*, Oxford: Oxford University Press.

Sturges, S. (1889) 'Doctors and Nurses', *The Nursing Record*, 28 March, p. 198.

Summers, A. (1979) 'A Home from Home: women's philanthropic work in the nineteenth century', in S. Burman (ed.) *Fit Work for Women*, London: Croom Helm, pp. 33–63.

Summers, A. (1988) *Angels and Citizens: British women as military nurses, 1854–1914*, London: Routledge and Kegan Paul.

Summers, A. (1989) 'The Mysterious Demise of Sarah Gamp: the domiciliary nurse and her detractors *c.*1830–1860', *Victorian Studies* 32 (spring), pp. 365–86.

Summers, A. (1991) 'The Costs and Benefits of Caring: nursing charities *c.*1830–1860', in J. Barry and C. Jones (eds) *Medicine and Charity before the Welfare State*, London: Routledge, pp. 133–48.

Summers, A. (2000) *Female Lives, Moral States: women, religion and public life in Britain 1800–1930*, London: Threshold Press.

Sweet, H. (2007) 'Establishing Connections, Restoring Relationships: Exploring the history of nursing in Britain', *Gender and History* 9 (3), pp. 565–80.

Sweet, H. and Dougal, R. (2008) *Community Nursing and Primary Care in Twentieth-Century Britain*, London: Routledge.

Tamboukou, M. (2000) 'Of Other Spaces: women's colleges at the turn of the century', *Gender Place and Culture* 7 (3), pp. 247–63.

Taylor, J. (1997) 'The Ladies Committee of the Women's Hospital, Castlegate, Nottingham 1880–1900', *International History of Nursing Journal* 2 (4), pp. 38–47.

Thompson F.M.L. (1988) *The Rise of Respectable Society: a social history of Victorian Britain 1830–1900*, London: Fontana Press.

Tiller, K. (1998) *English Local History: the state of the art*, Cambridge: Cambridge University Board of Continuing Education.

Tosh, J. (2006) *The Pursuit of History* (4th edition), Harlow: Pearson Education.

Trudgill, E. (1976) *Madonnas and Magdalens: the origins and development of Victorian sexual attitudes*, London: Heinemann.

Tusan, M.E. (2000) 'Not the Ordinary Victorian Charity: the Society for Promoting Employment for Women Archive', *History Workshop Journal* 49, pp. 220–30.

Vallone L. (1995) *Discipline of Virtue: girls' culture in the eighteenth and nineteenth centuries*, New Haven, CT: Yale University Press.

Versluysen, M. (1980) 'Old Wives Tales? Women healers in English history', in C. Davies (ed.) *Rewriting Nursing History*, London: Croom Helm, pp. 175–99.

Vicinus, M. (1985) *Independent Women: work and community for single women 1850–1920*, London: Virago.

Vickery, A. (1998) 'Golden Age to Separate Spheres? A review of the categories and chronology of English women's history', in P. Sharpe (ed.) *Women's Work: the English experience, 1860–1914*, London: Arnold, pp. 294–331.

Vickery, M.B. (2000) *Buildings for Bluestockings: the architecture and social history of women's colleges in late Victorian England*, London: University of Delaware Press.

Waddington, K. (1995) 'The Nursing Dispute at Guy's 1879–1880', *Social History of Medicine*, 8, pp. 211–30.

Waddington, K. (1996) 'Grasping Attitude: charity and hospital finance in late Victorian London', in M. Daunton (ed.) *Charity, Self Interest and Welfare in the English Past*, London: UCL Press, pp. 181–202.

Waddington, K. (2000) *Charity and the London Hospitals 1850–1898*, Woodbridge: Royal Historical Society, Boydell Press.

Waddington, K. (2003) 'Subscribing to a Democracy: management and voluntary ideology of the London hospitals 1850–1900', *English Historical Review* 118 (476), pp. 357–79.

Warren, M. (2000) *A Chronology of State Medicine, Public Health, Welfare and Related Services in Britain: 1066–1999*, London: Faculty of Public Health Medicine, Royal College of Physicians of the United Kingdom. Online. Available at www.fphm.org.uk/resources/atoz/r_chronology_of_state_medicine.pdf (accessed on 22 August 2009).

Webb, R.K. (2006) 'Harriet Martineau (1802–1876)', *Oxford Dictionary of National Biography*, Oxford: Oxford University Press. Online. Available at www.oxforddnb.com/view/article/18228 (accessed 14 December 2006);

Weekshaw, C. and Radford, W.A. (1897) *A Text-Book of Nursing*, London: Edward Arnold.

Weir, R. (2000) 'Medical and Nursing Education in the Nineteenth Century: comparisons and comments', *International History of Nursing Journal* 5 (2), pp. 42–7.

West, C. (1854) *How to Nurse Sick Children: intended especially as a help to the nurses at the Hospital for Sick Children*, London: Longman, Brown, Green and Longmans.

Whitaker, W. (1973) *The Victorian and Edwardian Shopworker: the struggle to obtain better conditions and a half-holiday*, Newton Abbott: David and Charles.

White, R. (1978) *Social Change and the Development of the Nursing Profession: a study of the Poor Law nursing service, 1848–1948*, London: H. Kimpton.

Wildman, S. (1999) 'The Development of Nursing at the General Hospital, Birmingham 1779–1919', *International History of Nursing Journal* 4 (3), pp. 20–8.

Wildman, S. (2003) 'The Development of Nurse Training in the Birmingham Teaching Hospitals 1869–1957', *International History of Nursing Journal* 7 (3), pp. 56–65.

Wildman, S. (2006) 'First Generation Nurses: the careers of trained working-class women, 1860–1900', presented at the Third Annual History of Nursing Conference: Race Class and Gender: the evolution of the modern nursing culture, 14 November 2006, London.

Wildman, S. (2007) 'Changes in Hospital Nursing in the West Midlands, 1841–1901', in J. Reinarz (ed.) *Medicine and Society in the Midlands*, Birmingham: Midland History Occasional Publications, pp. 98–114.

Wildman, S. (2009) ' "Nurses for all Classes": home nursing in England 1860–1900', *Medizin Gesellschaft und Geschichte* (Medicine, Society and History, Yearbook of the Institute for the History of Medicine at Robert Bosch Institution, Stuttgart), pp. 47–62.

Williams, K. (1980) 'From Sarah Gamp to Florence Nightingale', in C. Davies (ed.) *Rewriting Nursing History*, London: Croom Helm, pp. 41–75.

Witz, A. (1992) *Professions and Patriarchy*, London: Routledge.

Wood, C. (1888) Letter, *The Hospital*, 18 February, p. 350.

Wood, C. (1894) 'Three Aspects of Nursing Work', *Nursing Notes*, 1 May, pp. 54–5.

Wood, C. (1897) 'Private Nursing', *Nursing Notes*, 1 May, p. 60.

Woodham-Smith, C. (1950) *Florence Nightingale*, London: Constable.

Woodward, J. (1974) *To Do the Sick No Harm: a study of the British voluntary hospital system to 1875*, London: Routledge and Kegan Paul.

World Roots Website (n.d.) Online. Available at www.worldroots.com (accessed on 24 December 2006).

Wright, D. (1996) 'The Dregs of Society? Occupational patterns of male asylum attendants in Victorian England', *International History of Nursing Journal* 1 (4), pp. 5–19.

Yeo, G. (1995) *Nursing at Bart's: a history of nursing service and nurse education at St Bartholomew's Hospital, London*, London: St Bartholomew and Princess Alexandra and Newham College of Nursing and Midwifery.

Young, A. (2008) ' "Entirely a woman's question"? Class, Gender, and the Victorian Nurse', *Journal of Victorian Culture* 13 (1), pp 18–41.

Index

Printed and bound by CPI Group (UK) Ltd, Croydon, CR0 4YY

04/11/2024

01783488-0001